Color and Power
Doppler Sonography

Color and Power Doppler Sonography

A Teaching File

R. BROOKE JEFFREY, JR.

Professor of Radiology
Chief of Abdominal Imaging
Stanford University Medical Center

PHILIP W. RALLS

Professor of Radiology
Los Angeles County and
University of Southern California Medical Center

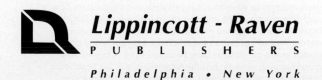

Lippincott - Raven
PUBLISHERS

Philadelphia • New York

Acquisitions Editor: James Ryan
Developmental Editor: Mary Beth Murphy
Manufacturing Manager: Dennis Teston
Production Manager: Larry Bernstein
Production Editor: Liane Carita
Cover Designer: Karen Quigley
Indexer: Pilar Wyman
Compositor: Maryland Composition
Printer: Toppan Printing Co.

Printed in Singapore

9 8 7 6 5 4 3 2 1

Library of Congress Cataloging-in-Publication Data

Jeffrey, R. Brooke.
    Color and power doppler sonography : a teaching file / R. Brooke
Jeffrey, Jr., Philip W. Ralls.
      p. cm.
    Includes bibliographical references and index.
    ISBN 0-397-51779-3 (alk. paper)
    1. Doppler ultrasonography.   I. Ralls, Philip W. (Philip
Whitney), 1948–   . II. Title.
    [DNLM: 1. Ultrasonography, Doppler, Color. WN 208 J46c 1997]
RC78.7.U4J44 1997
616.07'543—dc21
DCLM/DLC
for Library of Congress

To Renee, Colin, Whitney, Stefanie, Catherine, Elizabeth, and Luke with love.

Contents

Preface

Color and power Doppler sonography represent important technical advances for noninvasive vascular imaging. The ability to rapidly survey an anatomic region and delineate vascular flow patterns without the use of contrast agents is a powerful clinical tool. Many pathologic conditions are characterized by abnormal flow states. Flow may be increased in tumors, inflammation, and arteriovenous shunts. Flow may be decreased or absent in ischemia, infarction, or vascular occlusion. The documentation of normal flow may also be of considerable clinical value in excluding the previously mentioned disorders. The purpose of this book is twofold. First, it is to review the basic principles underlying the physics and technical aspects of color and power Doppler. Second, it is to illustrate the broad spectrum of clinical utility of color flow imaging in routine practice. It is our hope that this book will be a useful clinically oriented review highlighting the diagnostic value of color and power Doppler.

Acknowledgment

We would like to acknowledge Kevin Murphy and Betty Hemphill for their patience and support.

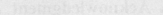

Color and Power
Doppler Sonography

SECTION 1

Principles, Pitfalls, and Practical Hints

INTRODUCTION

Color flow sonography (CFS) passively and automatically displays color-coded flow information superimposed on all or a selected portion of the grayscale image. Flow is revealed in real time within the selected region of interest. This is quite different from conventional spectral Doppler (single-sample volume Doppler, sometimes known as "duplex Doppler"). Spectral Doppler does not reveal flow automatically. The operator must actively seek flow by moving a small sensitive area (known as the sample volume or range gate) over the image. If the person scanning does not interrogate an area, flow will not be detected; unexpected flow will be missed. Thus, color flow sonography provides flow information from a large area faster and with less operator dependence than does spectral Doppler.

Spectral Doppler is useful when detailed quantitative information about flow velocities is important (e.g., carotid imaging). Color flow sonography facilitates fast and accurate spectral Doppler

sample volume placement in these applications. For example, color flow sonography can quickly detect the region of highest velocity in a stenotic artery or reveal an intrarenal artery that is invisible on grayscale. Color flow sonography then quickly and accurately guides placement of the spectral Doppler sample volume.

Color flow sonography is used alone when flow detection or global anatomic information about blood flow is needed to make a diagnosis. Color flow sonography's capability of providing a global view of flow in real time minimizes the chance of missing flow in an unexpected area and facilitates comparison of flow in different anatomic locations. Color flow sonography has the advantage of displaying both flow and anatomic information in a real-time image. The real-time color flow image is much easier to understand than a combined grayscale/spectral duplex Doppler display.

BASIC PRINCIPLES

In color flow sonography, both flow direction and frequency shift (proportional to flow velocity) are color coded. Usually, the colors red and blue are used to represent flow direction toward or away from the ultrasound beam (transducer) (Fig. 1). It is important to remember that color Doppler sonography displays average Doppler frequency shift, not true angle-corrected velocity. In the qualitative flow images produced with real-time color Doppler sonography, mean frequency shift is proportional to flow velocity. Color Doppler images generally do a good job of displaying relative blood flow velocities within the area imaged.

Mean frequency shift (proportional to flow velocity) is often displayed as a difference in color saturation. The whiter, paler colors (less color saturation) correspond to faster flow velocity (greater mean frequency shifts). The deeper reds and blues (more saturated colors) correspond to slower velocities (lower mean frequency shifts) (Fig. 2). Another type of display uses different colors (hues) to code for velocity/frequency shift. This display is called a hue map (color-change or "rainbow" map) (Fig. 3). It is easier to detect color Doppler aliasing (see the Artifacts section) on a hue (color change) map image than on a color saturation map image. With most systems, the user has a choice of color flow maps. Power Doppler techniques do not show flow direction or velocity information (see the Power Doppler Techniques section). Power Doppler images generally use displays that reflect the energy/power of the flow rather than direction or velocity.

Color flow sonography differs significantly from spectral Doppler. With spectral Doppler, the small sample volume is interrogated many times—as many as 200—for each image line. This results in a comprehensive display of the entire

spectrum of Doppler frequency shifts. Not only is the peak frequency shift displayed, but so are all others. Since color flow sonography must display flow information and a grayscale image in real time, the information contained in each image line is necessarily more limited. Each real-time image line is derived from relatively few samples (typically 8 to 16) from each scan line (view). This is many fewer samples per line than spectral Doppler. Thus, as a practical matter, color flow sonography can display only mean frequency shift (proportional to velocity) and variance (roughly corre-

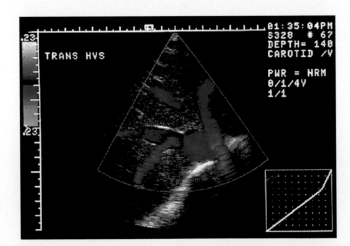

FIG. 1. Color coding of flow direction: transverse color flow image of the liver. Normal hepatic veins with blood flow into the inferior vena cava. Typically, flow toward the transducer is coded *red*. Flow away from the transducer is generally coded *blue*.

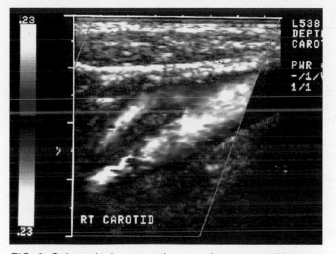

FIG. 2. Color velocity saturation map image: carotid artery system. With this flow map, the more saturated, *deeper colors* represent lower-frequency shifts (corresponding to slower velocity) near the vessel walls. The *whiter colors* represent higher-frequency shifts, which correspond to flow velocity in the center of the vessel. Aliasing is not detected in this image.

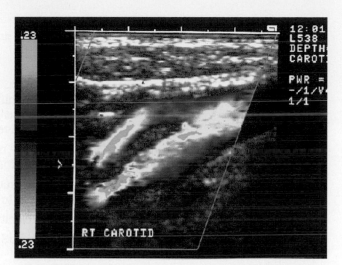

FIG. 3. Color velocity hue map image: carotid artery system. This is the same image as Fig. 2, using a different flow map. With this flow map, different frequency shifts are displayed as different colors. Note that the slower velocities (small frequency shifts) near the vessel wall are *deep red*. The more rapid, midstream velocities are coded as *orange* or *yellow*. Aliasing (*green* and *blue* areas) is readily detected in this color-change map image. Hue maps are synonymous with color-change or "rainbow" maps.

sponding to spectral broadening). Spectral Doppler displays the entire range of frequency shifts, but only within the small area of the range gate. In essence, color flow sonography provides less complete flow information, but with the added benefit of providing a more global and easily understood flow image.

FACTORS INFLUENCING THE FLOW IMAGE

In the context of color Doppler sonography, the Doppler effect refers to the frequency shift observed when sound is reflected from a moving target: red blood cell aggregates. From the Doppler equation (Fig. 4), we see that the Doppler shift is influenced by the following factors:

1. The frequency of the ultrasound beam (f) used to interrogate flow
2. The angle of the ultrasound beam to flow direction (θ)
3. The velocity of flowing red blood cell aggregates (V)

For clinical Doppler sonography, the primary scatterers (aggregates of red blood cells) are much smaller than the wavelength of the insonating beam. Because of this size relationship, the intensity of the backscattered echoes is governed by Rayleigh–Tyndall scattering. This means that the signal intensity varies with the fourth power of the insonant beam frequency. Thus, if the Doppler frequency doubles (e.g., from 2 to 4 MHz), signal intensity increases 16 times. Conversely, lowering beam frequency (e.g., from 4 to 2 MHz) results in one-16th the signal (Fig. 5). Obviously, higher-frequency (5 to 10 MHz) transducers are more sensitive in scanning superficial flow because more signal results. Another advantage of high frequency is better spatial resolution.

The main disadvantage of high-frequency transducers is poor tissue penetration. High-frequency beams are quickly attenuated (Fig. 6). Frequency effects are much more important for Doppler sonography than for grayscale imaging. The Doppler frequency shift signal is many times fainter than the echoes used to produce grayscale images. As a practical matter, high-frequency Doppler (5 to 7 MHz) simply can't penetrate tissue well enough to obtain good flow information deeper than 6 cm in most patients. At that depth, lower frequency (2 to 3 MHz) is preferred for its better tissue penetration. There is a trade-off between tissue penetration (low frequency) and higher Doppler shifts (high frequency). When superficial organs or vessels are scanned, tissue penetration is not a problem; high-frequency transducers are better to use because they yield greater frequency shifts. In abdominal and other deep Doppler applications, however, the need for adequate tissue penetration is predominant. Obviously, if sound does not penetrate deeply enough, flow cannot be displayed. Thus, in many applications, penetration/attenuation effects predominate, and lower-frequency transducers should be used even at the cost of lower echo intensity. In some patients, trying both higher and lower frequency may be necessary to optimize flow imaging. With some modern high-bandwidth transducers, several different Doppler frequencies can be produced, allowing more flexibility without having to change transducers (Figs. 7A and B).

Lower scan angles produce larger Doppler shifts. Maximum Doppler frequency shift occurs when blood is flowing

$$\text{Frequency (fd)} = \frac{2\ f\ V\ \text{cosine}\ \theta}{C}$$

Where:

$F(fd)$ = Doppler shift frequency
(the difference between the transmitted
and received frequencies)

f = Frequency of incident US beam
(emitted from transducer)

C = Speed of sound in the body
(assumed to be 1540 m/s)

V = RBC Velocity

θ = Angle of US beam to Flow direction

FIG. 4. The Doppler equation.

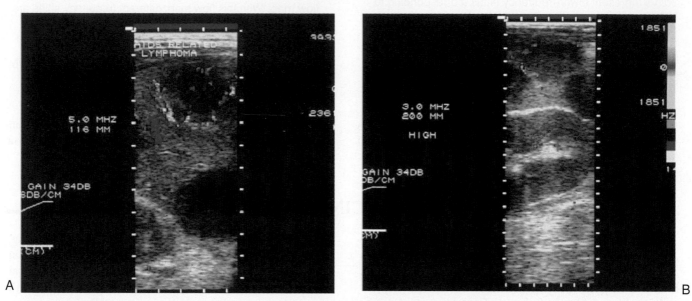

FIG. 5. AIDS-related lymphoma of the liver: enhanced flow with higher frequency. When the tumor is imaged at 3 MHz, much less flow is displayed. The greater frequency shift obtained in superficial flow with higher insonant frequency explains the difference.

directly toward or away from the ultrasound beam ($\theta = 0°$ or $180°$). Thus, scanning as close as is possible to $0°$ will optimize sensitivity and minimize ambiguity in flow direction. Conversely, as the scan angle approaches $90°$, frequency shift decreases, sensitivity decreases, and directional ambiguity increases (Figs. 8A and B). At $90°$, cosine $\theta = 0$. Hence, blood flowing perpendicularly to the ultrasound beam (generally, parallel to the transducer face) will not be displayed, because no Doppler shift is generated (Fig. 9). Because flow is not truly uniform in any vessel, some color-coded flow may be displayed, even in vessels that are apparently perpendicular to the beam (Figs. 8A and B). Blood flowing at uniform velocity in a vessel is displayed as different colors when imaged at different angles. Thus, blood flow in a tortuous vessel will be represented by several different colors in the same image, with a black line representing the re-

gion of flow direction change (Fig. 10). The black line occurs because the high-pass filter ("wall filter") eliminates the very low frequency shifts that occur at and near a $90°$ scan angle. Sector and curved linear transducers produce divergent scan lines—their displays are wider in the far field than in the near field. Blood flow in a vessel parallel to the transducer face of a sector or curved linear transducer will be displayed as red on one side of the vessel and blue on the other, separated by an intervening black line (Fig. 11). These color changes occur because the divergent scan lines intersect flow at different angles from one side of the image to the other.

The velocity of blood flow is the most important parameter influencing the Doppler frequency shift. The purpose of color flow sonography is, after all, to display blood flow. Color flow sonography images, which are not angle corrected, display frequency shift, not flow velocity. Thus, color

4

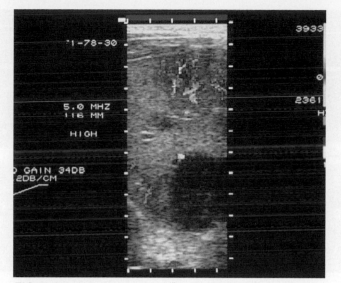

FIG. 6. HIV lymphoma, focal liver masses: inadequate tissue penetration to display deeper lesion. Flow is shown in the more superficial hepatic lesion, but tissue penetration is insufficient to display flow adequately in a deeper lesion, even though both are identical histologically. A lower frequency is often needed to provide adequate tissue penetration for color flow images.

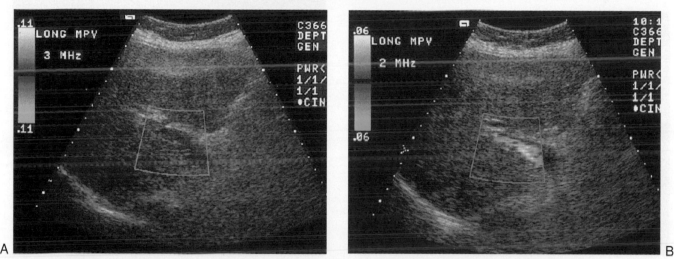

A

B

FIG. 7. Better tissue penetration with lower frequency: enhanced flow sensitivity. A: A longitudinal image of the main portal vein obtained at 3 MHz shows only a small amount of flow within the portal vein, suggesting partial portal vein thrombosis. B: A 2-MHz color Doppler image reveals flow throughout the vessel. Tissue penetration provided by low frequency is often the key to visualizing flow in deep vessels. The shift to a lower Doppler frequency was achieved using the same transducer. Some modern high-bandwidth transducers can transmit two or more different Doppler frequencies, lessening the need to change transducers.

Doppler images are really "average frequency shift" displays, not a map of actual, angle-corrected velocity. This ordinarily causes no clinical difficulty. Color Doppler images generally do a good job of displaying relative blood flow velocities within the area imaged.

Beam characteristics have an important impact on Doppler ultrasound. A wide, relatively unfocused beam profile with a long pulse length is best for Doppler. An unfocused beam allows uniform power input into the target area (usually a vessel) and thus produces a more uniform frequency response. Narrowly focused beams, typically used for grayscale imaging, may result in random variability of the Doppler shift. With a tightly focused, narrow beam, the Doppler shift may be more related to suboptimal beam characteristics rather than the actual flow velocity.

Optimal Doppler sonography and grayscale imaging have conflicting requirements. Grayscale imaging is best performed with a 90° scan angle, a narrowly focused beam,

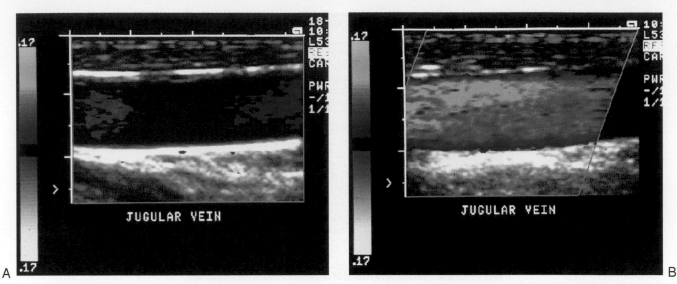

A   B

FIG. 8. Jugular vein: flow ambiguity at a 90° scan angle. In the Doppler equation, the cosine of θ at 90° is 0. Thus, little flow is displayed at scan angles of ~90°. Conversely, the lower the angle, the better are the color Doppler images. A: In this image, where the scan angle is ~90°, little flow is displayed. The few frequency shifts displayed are ambiguous and confusing. B: In this image, the scan angle is sufficiently less than 90° (indicated by the slant of the *color box*) to enable an unambiguous display of the direction of flow, which fills the entire vessel.

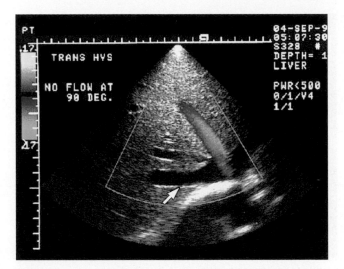

FIG. 9. Hepatic veins entering the inferior vena cava: no flow at 90°. Note the robust display of flow from the middle hepatic vein into the inferior vena cava. Flow is shown well because the low scan angle (~0°) results in more Doppler signal. The right hepatic vein (*arrow*) is being imaged at a nearly perpendicular angle (~90°). At this angle, no flow is detected. Angle effects are important. Imaging at a low scan angle is necessary to obtain optimal flow sensitivity.

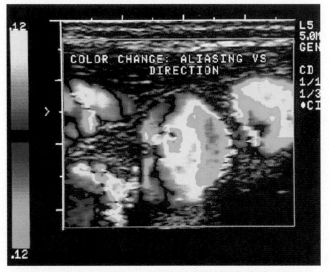

FIG. 10. Superficial abdominal collateral vein: aliasing. Multiple color changes related to aliasing and true directional change are noted within this vessel. Color-change-related aliasing is easy to detect because the color transition occurs between frequency shifts representing the highest velocities in opposite directions (yellow and green). There is no intervening black line. True color flow direction changes are displayed as transitions between the lowest frequency shifts (red and blue), separated by a black line.

and short ultrasound pulses (to optimize spatial resolution); whereas Doppler shift is maximal at 0°, and frequency response is most uniform when a relatively unfocused beam and a long pulse length are used. Frequency requirements also differ. Higher frequency is generally better for grayscale, where spatial resolution needs predominate. With Doppler, penetration is often crucial, and lower frequency achieves better results. These conflicting requirements make it easy to appreciate the engineering challenges involved in producing an effective real-time color Doppler

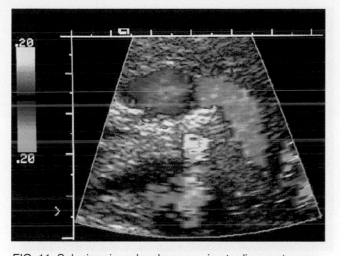

FIG. 11. Splenic vein: color change owing to divergent scan lines. All sector and curved linear transducers produce divergent scan lines. In this image, the splenic vein is largely parallel to the transducer face, so divergent scan lines intersect flow at different angles. In this circumstance, flow will be displayed as *red* on one side of the vessel and *blue* on the other. The intervening *black line* between the blue- and red-coded flows represents the region in which the wall filter eliminates very low frequency shifts at or near a 90° scan angle.

sonographic system. Several approaches to this problem have been used in commercial instruments.

Successful clinical color Doppler systems (CDS) require advanced technology. Necessary features include (a) flexible and fast beam-forming capabilities, (b) powerful computer processing, and (c) superb signal detection and processing. Because of these requirements, most color flow sonography is performed with either phased-array or linear-array transducers, because these have a sufficiently large number of elements and channels to allow appropriate beam forming. The three basic processing approaches to color flow sonography are (a) autocorrelation CDS, (b) linear multi-

gated CDS, and (c) moving target indicator CDS (cross-correlation).

Autocorrelation color Doppler compares three or more (typically 8 to 12) samples of the same view (scan line) for each real-time image frame. The data from the 8 to 12 samples are compared and all stationary echoes are eliminated, leaving only the Doppler-shifted echoes. The images are produced with information from these moving, Doppler-shifted echoes. Autocorrelation yields phase and frequency information that is used to create color Doppler flow images. The autocorrelation signal has another feature: amplitude. Power Doppler images are produced from the amplitude information. Two entirely separate beams are formed for flow and grayscale imaging—a more focused beam for grayscale and an angled, less focused beam for Doppler. Autocorrelation is the method that most manufacturers have chosen to produce color flow images.

The linear multigated technique involves acquiring an entire line of sample volumes at more or less the same time. Multiple gates are almost simultaneously received and, in essence, Doppler shifts are gathered from an entire scan line broken up into individual sample volumes. Grayscale and Doppler images are produced from the same scan information. This technique can have excellent sensitivity, but is complex and computationally demanding. Trade-offs between grayscale and flow image quality must be made. Autocorrelation is faster and has better spectral resolution than does the linear multigated technique.

Time-of-flight techniques (cross-correlation) directly measure the actual distance that reflectors move, with a direct calculation of flow velocity. Other techniques for displaying blood flow on ultrasound images are possible. Each approach to flow imaging has its own theoretical advantages and disadvantages. From the radiologist's perspective, clinical performance is the only important criterion. The success of color flow sonography systems generally depends more on engineering considerations than on the technique used to produce the image.

POWER DOPPLER TECHNIQUES

Autocorrelation yields phase and frequency information (used to create color Doppler flow images) and amplitude. Amplitude can also be used to create flow images—that is, images with characteristics that are different from traditional phase/frequency (color Doppler) images. Amplitude is integrated to reflect the power/energy of the autocorrelation signal. Various names have been given to this type of color flow imaging: power Doppler, color amplitude imaging, color power, or color energy Doppler. We will use power Doppler because that is the term used by Prof. Jonathan Rubin (University of Michigan), who popularized this technique.

The most important benefit of power Doppler imaging is improved flow sensitivity. Modern color Doppler is capable

of displaying intrarenal flow in vessels that are invisible on grayscale images (Figs. 12A and B). With power Doppler, noise is much less intrusive than on conventional phase/frequency color Doppler images. With power Doppler, noise is displayed as low power, whereas phase/frequency color Doppler noise may have any frequency shift. Frequency noise, then, may cause very large frequency shifts. These deceptive, noise-related frequency shifts can result in color artifacts that seriously degrade conventional color Doppler flow images (Figs. 13A and B). Low noise means better signal-to-noise ratio—this translates into better flow sensitivity. As a practical matter, power Doppler images can be amplified 10 to 15 dB more than autocorrelation phase/frequency

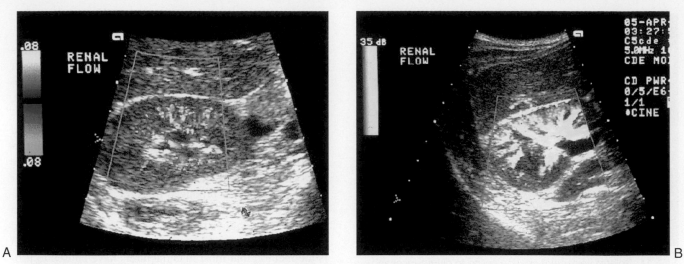

FIG. 12. A and B: Intrarenal flow. A is color Doppler image and B is power Doppler image. Image shows more flow. Intralobular arteries and "parenchymal blush" are shown out to the renal capsule. This type of image is possible because of the increased sensitivity to flow available with power Doppler.

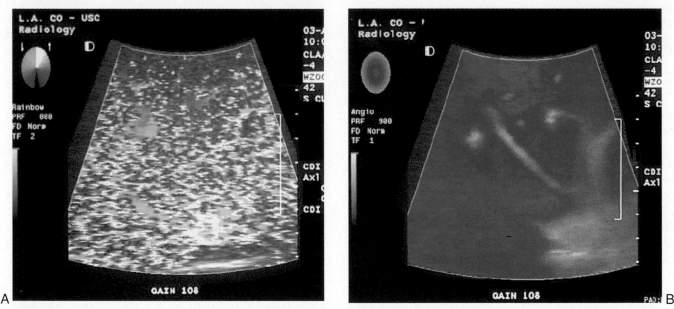

FIG. 13. Hepatic veins entering the inferior vena cava: noise is more distracting with color Doppler than with power Doppler. The superior signal-to-noise characteristics of power Doppler images enable better images to be obtained at high gain than do conventional phase frequency color Doppler images. Both the color Doppler sonogram (A) and the power Doppler sonogram (B) were performed at comparable gain (amplification) settings. A: Noise is much more obtrusive in the color Doppler image, essentially destroying any diagnostic content. B: In this power Doppler image, noise is displayed as low power (*blue* and *purple*). The flow in the hepatic veins and inferior vena cava (coded *orange*) is clearly noted.

color Doppler images before noise becomes intrusive. Consequently, with power Doppler flow imaging, one can scan at higher gain settings without destroying the image with artifact.

Other characteristics of current power Doppler flow imaging include the absence of directional information, the absence of aliasing, and relative insensitivity to angle of flow. This means flow can be imaged better at scan angles nearer 90° (perpendicular to flow) than with color Doppler (Figs. 14A and B). The lack of aliasing is not particularly advantageous, especially as flow direction cannot currently be displayed by power Doppler flow imaging.

The enhanced sensitivity from power Doppler flow imaging is useful in many scanning circumstances. One hope is that these techniques will eventually provide a parenchymal flow image in many organs. Such images are routinely possible with current technology in the high-flow kidney (Fig. 15). Improved sensitivity and the addition of contrast agents may enable parenchymal contrast en-

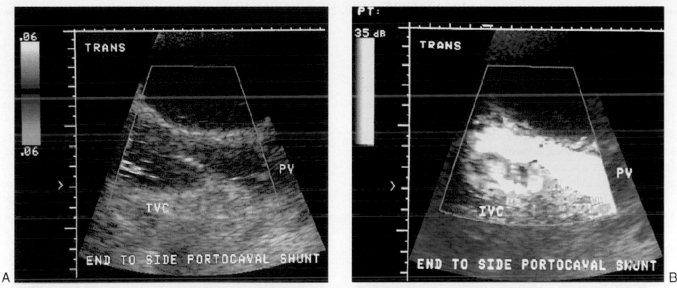

FIG. 14. End-to-side portocaval shunt: flow seen better with power Doppler. The patient had portal hypertension that caused bleeding esophageal varices, so an end-to-side portocaval shunt was performed to decompress the portal venous system. A: This transverse color Doppler sonogram shows very little flow in the region of the anastomosis of the shunt. Presumably, the color Doppler image revealed little flow because the angle of insonation to flow is ~90°. B: This power Doppler sonogram in the same region clearly shows that the shunt is widely patent. Power Doppler's better sensitivity at flow angles ~90° provided important diagnostic information in this case.

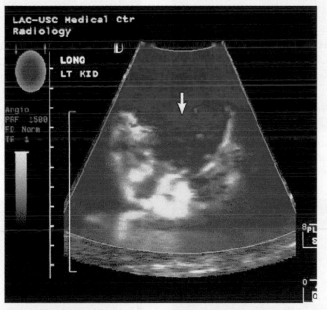

FIG. 15. Renal infarct: flow void with power Doppler. A transverse power Doppler image of the left kidney reveals a clear-cut flow void, representing a renal infarct (*arrow*). Decreased flow was difficult to appreciate on the color Doppler image (not shown).

hancement in the liver, spleen, and other organs. One current disadvantage of power Doppler is that it is more susceptible to motion artifact than is color Doppler, generally because higher frame averaging is used than with color Doppler. "Flash" artifacts, caused by moving soft tissue, are very pronounced because moving soft tissue has much higher amplitude than does flowing blood. Power Doppler's slow frame rate can make it difficult to track flow in a vessel in real time, especially when patients cannot hold their breath.

9

Doppler sonography is easier in superficial vessels and in vessels with high-volume, high-velocity flow—the carotid artery, for example. Deeper vessels, small vessels, and vessels with slow flow present a challenge to the engineer and clinical practitioner alike. Many factors are important when flow sensitivity is a problem. To ensure good acoustic access, which is an absolute prerequisite, the examiner must often try several patient positions, acoustic windows, and transducers. Remember that a scan angle as close to 0° as possible will maximize sensitivity to flow.

There is a trade-off between the higher echo intensity provided by high frequency, and the need for tissue penetration provided by lower frequency. In superficial applications, higher frequency is generally best (Figs. 16A and B). In all other situations, tissue penetration is usually the dominant requirement, and lower frequency improves sensitivity (Figs. 17A and B). The best policy to improve flow sensitivity is to increase frequency for superficial scans and decrease frequency for deeper applications. In the 4- to 6-cm-depth range, the sonographer may have to try both higher frequency and lower frequency to determine which is better.

Once good acoustic access at a low scan angle and the correct frequency have been found, other parameters must be optimized (Tables 1 and 2). The highest allowable power output

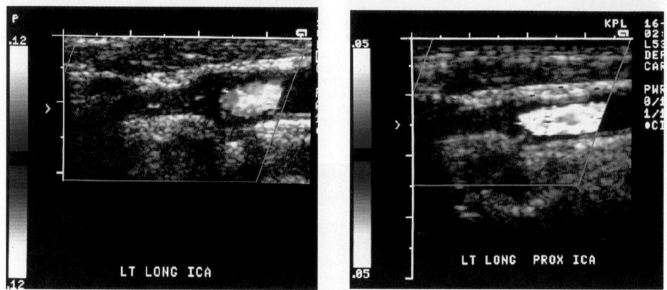

FIG. 16. High-grade carotid stenosis: higher frequency yields better sensitivity. When scanning superficial structures, higher-frequency Doppler is advantageous. A: This color Doppler image obtained at 5 MHz suggests complete obstruction of the internal carotid artery. B: This 7-MHz image shows flow through a high-grade carotid stenosis.

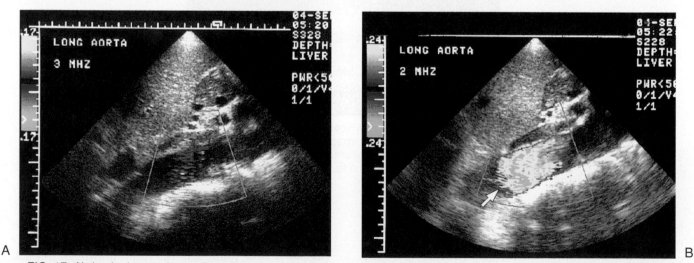

FIG. 17. Abdominal aorta: better flow display with lower frequency. When scanning deeper structures, low-frequency tissue penetration needs are predominant. Although the 3-MHz image (A) shows some flow within the abdominal aorta, an image obtained at 2 MHz (B) shows the flow to much better advantage. Some aliasing is present (*arrow*). The higher-frequency image (A) demonstrates suboptimal tissue penetration.

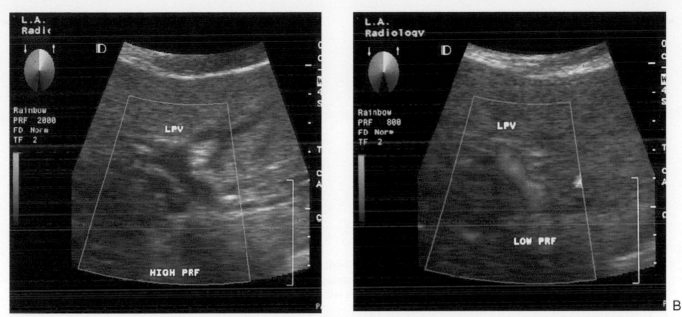

FIG. 18. Enhanced sensitivity with lower PRF: decreasing PRF improves signal-to-noise characteristics and thus enhances sensitivity. A: A high PRF color Doppler sonogram of the left portal vein reveals poor flow sensitivity. B: When the PRF is lowered, a more robust flow display results.

TABLE 1. *High sensitivity scanning: initial steps*

Parameter		Adjustment
Acoustic access	→	Optimize
Frequency	→	High vs low (penetration)
Scan angle	→	As close to 0° as possible
Power output	→	Maximum allowable
Color gain	→	Increase to near noise floor
Focal zone depth	→	Set depth at area of interest

TABLE 2. *High-sensitivity scanning: fine-tuning steps*

Parameter		Adjustment
Color priority	→	Prioritize flow display
Pulse repetition frequency	→	Decrease
Wall filter	→	Decrease
Sample volume (gate) size	→	Increase
Ensemble length*	→	Increase
Color-box width	→	Decrease
Color-frame averaging	→	Increase

* Also called "packet size" or "dwell time."

should be used. Note that energy deposition with color flow imaging is much less than with spectral Doppler. The maximum signal amplification (color "gain") that does not introduce artifact is best. A low pulse repetition frequency (PRF) (Figs. 18A and B and 19A and B) and low wall filter (Figs. 20A and B) improve sensitivity.

Decreasing PRF enhances sensitivity by improving signal-to-noise characteristics. Color flow autocorrelation images are formed by comparing 8 to 16 consecutive scan lines ("ensemble length" or "packet size"). If the PRF is decreased, the interval between pulses is increased. A longer time period is required to acquire the data for each image, which means the frequency shift is greater. Greater frequency shifts mean more signal. Low PRF images are, therefore, more sensitive to flow. The negative effects of low PRF include lower frame rates and increased susceptibility to motion artifact.

A moderate to high wall filter often eliminates diagnostically useful frequency shifts that arise from slowly flowing blood. An image acquired with a lower wall filter displays more low-frequency shifts—they are not filtered out. This enhances

overall color Doppler flow sensitivity, especially to slow flow.

Other features that increase signal-to-noise ratio should be employed to enhance sensitivity. A larger effective sample volume can do this. Increasing the number of samples per display line (called increased "ensemble length," "packet size," or "dwell time") or increasing frame averaging also improves the signal-to-noise ratio. A narrower color box may be useful for increasing line density and improving spatial resolution and possibly sensitivity. Many instruments can be adjusted to preferentially write color flow rather than grayscale for slowly moving reflectors—a color/grayscale priority control. All of these manipulations are associated with image trade-offs, generally decreased frame rate and increased artifact. Tables 1 and 2 summarize how to achieve some of the aforementioned goals.

Some machines use application-specific presets to get the examiner "in the ballpark" for specific indications. Nevertheless, optimal sensitivity color flow imaging usually requires some alteration from these presets. Power Doppler and spectral Doppler can also be used to detect flow more sensitively.

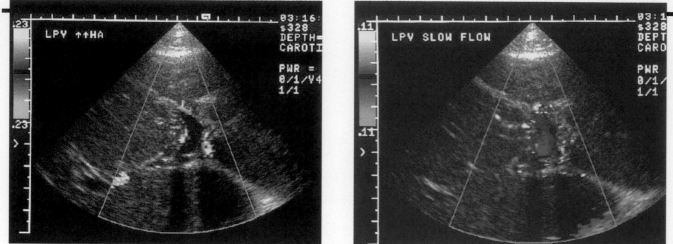

FIG. 19. Portal hypertension: flow reversal shown with low PRF. A: No flow is demonstrated within the left portal vein when a moderate PRF is employed. Note the prominent arteries and smaller vessels with severely aliased flow. A lower PRF enhances sensitivity. B: Abnormal reversed flow in the left portal vein (coded *blue*), indicative of severe portal hypertension, is clearly displayed.

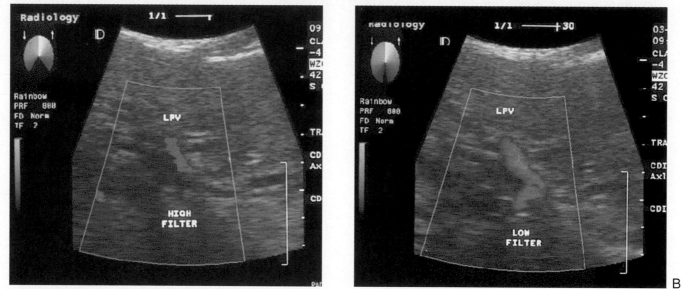

FIG. 20. Enhanced sensitivity with a lower wall filter. Transverse sonograms of the left portal vein show that a low wall filter (A) provides a better flow display than does a similar image obtained with a high wall filter (B). A moderate to high wall filter often eliminates diagnostically useful frequency shifts that arise from slowly flowing blood. An image acquired with a lower wall filter displays more low-frequency shifts—they are not filtered out. This enhances overall color Doppler flow sensitivity, especially to slow flow.

ARTIFACTS

Color flow sonography is susceptible to many of the same artifacts that occur with grayscale sonography. Artifacts may be related to electrical interference, equipment problems, or to the interaction of sound in tissue. We now address some artifacts that are potentially troubling on color flow sonographic images.

Mirror image artifacts occur when sound is reflected by strong reflectors and also bounces off interfaces within the structure imaged. The flow artifact appears as a mirror image of the real vessel, displayed at an apparently greater depth

than the actual vessel (Figs. 21 and 22), because the multiple reflections between the strong reflector and the vessel walls result in greater time of flight. Put another way, the flow is displayed deeper than its actual location because of the increased time it takes the echoes to return to the transducer, owing to the longer path that the sound has traveled.

Another potentially confusing artifact is color overwrite, which occurs most often when high-sensitivity scanning parameters are used. A hypoechoic or anechoic area is overwritten with color, falsely simulating flow. Moving soft tis-

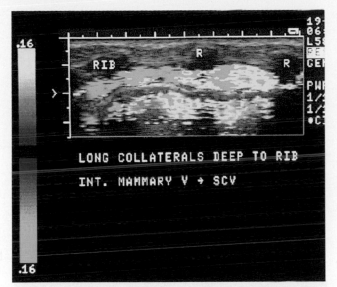

FIG. 21. Internal mammary portosystemic collateral: mirror-image artifact. This longitudinal image depicts flow in a portosystemic collateral in the internal mammary distribution. A mirror-image flow artifact is seen, deep to the actual vessel. Mirror-image artifacts occur when sound is reflected by strong, nearby reflectors and also bounces off interfaces within the structure itself. The mirror image is displayed in an apparently greater depth than the actual vessel because the multiple reflections result in greater time of flight.

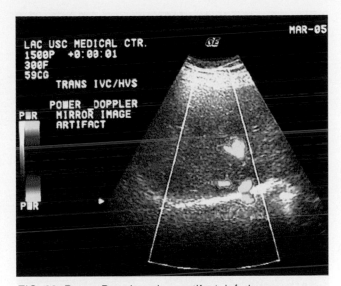

FIG. 22. Power Doppler mirror artifact: inferior vena cava and hepatic veins. A transverse power Doppler image near the dome of the liver shows flow in the inferior vena cava and two hepatic veins. Mirror-image reflections of these vessels are seen displayed deeper than the real vessels. Mirror-image artifacts occur when sound is reflected by strong reflectors—the diaphragm in this case—and also bounces off interfaces within the structure imaged.

sue (often caused by cardiac or respiratory motion) and slowly flowing blood may have similar frequency shifts. The color flow ultrasound system must determine whether to display grayscale or color for these relatively small frequency shifts. Soft tissue echo amplitude is much greater than that returning from flowing blood. This fact can be used to help distinguish moving soft tissue from blood flow. High-amplitude echoes are assumed to be moving tissue and are thus displayed as grayscale. Lower-amplitude echoes are assumed to be flowing blood and are displayed as color flow. Thus, a cyst or other low-echogenicity structure may be written falsely as color flow (Figs. 23A–D and 24A and B), while surrounding higher-echogenicity tissue is written as grayscale.

When the blood flow velocity is relatively high and a low PRF is used, aliasing may result. Put another way, aliasing occurs when there is an insufficient sampling rate (i.e., PRF is too low) to yield an unambiguous flow display. Aliasing in color Doppler displays may appear as a seemingly random mosaic of intermingled colors (severe aliasing) (Figs. 25A and B) or a mixture of the colors representing flow in both directions (mild aliasing) (Fig. 26).

Detecting severe aliasing presents no serious problem. Mild color aliasing can, however, simulate flow in a direction opposite to the true flow direction (Figs. 27A and B). Mild color aliasing can be distinguished from a change in flow direction. The key observation is whether there is a black line separating the colors in the transition. Color changes related to mild aliasing are easy to detect, because the color transition occurs between frequency shifts representing the highest velocities in opposite directions. There is no intervening black line. The color transition related to a true change in flow direction occurs between the colors representing the lowest frequency shifts, separated by an intervening black line. Multiple color changes related to aliasing and true directional change are noted within this vessel. Color-change-related aliasing is easy to detect because the color transition occurs between frequency shifts representing the highest velocities in opposite directions (yellow and green). There is no intervening black line (Fig. 10). True color flow direction changes are displayed as transitions between the lowest frequency shifts (red and blue), separated by a black line. The black line occurs where there are low-frequency shifts (incident angle ~90°)—so low that they are filtered out by the wall filter.

It is easier to detect mild color aliasing on color-change maps (hue or "rainbow") rather than on color saturation flow displays (Figs. 2 and 3). The transition in color saturation maps is displayed as white—no different from high-velocity, unaliased flow. In color-change maps, a color change enables easy identification. In abdominal imaging, aliasing may actually prove to be a useful artifact. For the frequencies generally used in abdominal imaging, arteries often have aliased flow. The slower flow present in veins may be unaliased. This can facilitate distinction of arteries from veins during the color real-time examination (Fig. 28).

Tissue hum, that is, vibration associated with high-velocity blood flow through arteriovenous fistulas and arteriovenous malformations, may appear as color-overwritten adja-

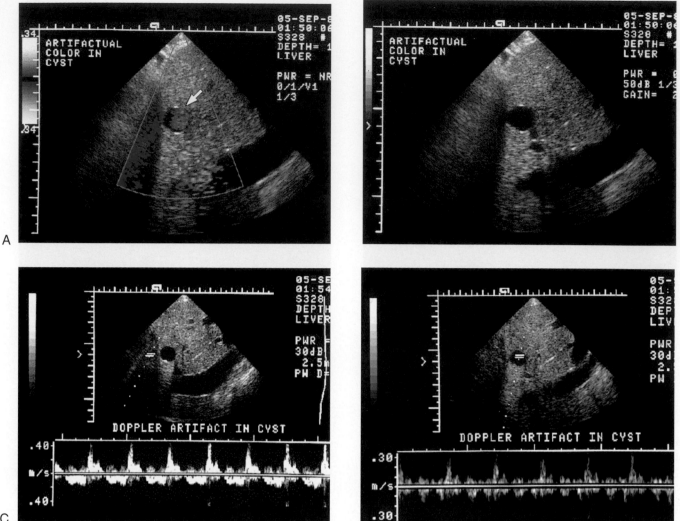

FIG. 23. Color-overwrite artifact in an hepatic cyst. A: This longitudinal color Doppler sonogram shows color displayed within an hepatic cyst (*arrow*). Some flash artifact is noted in the soft tissues near the cyst. B: This grayscale image shows classic findings for a cyst. Spectral Doppler is sometimes useful in sorting out color flow artifacts. In this instance, however, flow related to cardiac motion (C) is transmitted to the region of the cyst (D), so the spectral Doppler cannot definitively distinguish this artifact from actual flow. This cyst was confirmed with other imaging procedures, including computed tomography.

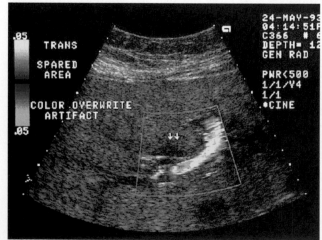

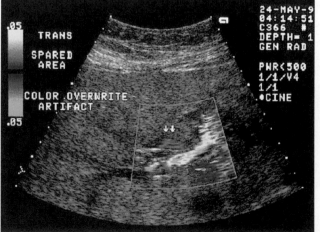

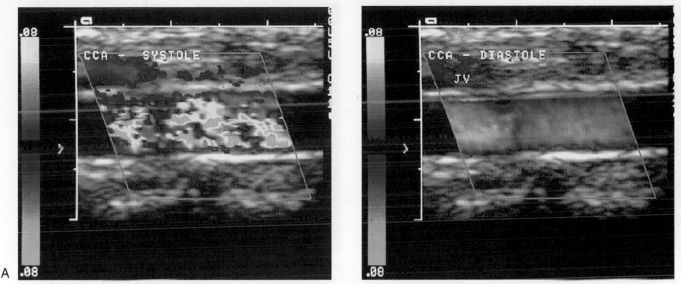

A   B

FIG. 25. Severe color Doppler aliasing: common carotid. A: When undersampling is extreme, color Doppler images display a random mosaic mixture of colors within the vessel. B: The slower flow in diastole results in adequate sampling, yielding an image displaying flow direction unambiguously.

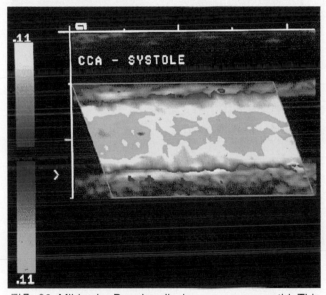

FIG. 26. Mild color Doppler aliasing: common carotid. This image of a common carotid artery obtained in systole shows midstream color Doppler aliasing. This is mild aliasing: the flows visualized do not "wrap around" many times, producing a mottled color mosaic (see Fig. 25). Mild aliasing is easy to detect on color-change map images, such as this one.

FIG. 24. Spared area, fatty liver: color-overwrite artifact. A: This transverse color Doppler sonogram near the region of the porta hepatis shows an hypoechoic area ventral to the portal vein. This appearance and location is typical for a spared area within a fatty liver. B: In another image, color is written into the nonvascular hypoechoic area, a color-overwrite artifact. With high-sensitivity settings, color flow can be written into areas that are not vessels when those areas have low-amplitude echoes (anechoic or hypoechoic).

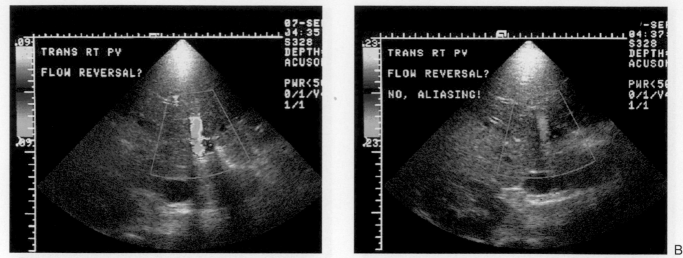

FIG. 27. A and B: Aliasing simulates flow reversal: right portal vein. These transverse images of the right portal vein obtained with relatively low PRF revealed *blue*-coded flows within the vessel. This color Doppler aliasing initially led to an erroneous diagnosis of flow reversal. Increasing the sampling rate showed that flow was normal, toward the periphery of the liver. The color transition between the highest frequency shifts, without an intervening black line, is the key to recognizing mild aliasing.

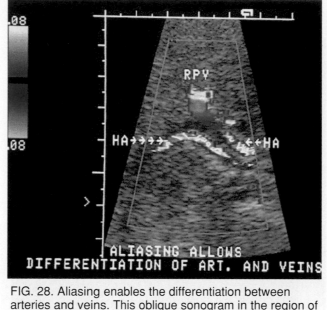

FIG. 28. Aliasing enables the differentiation between arteries and veins. This oblique sonogram in the region of the right portal vein shows unaliased hepatopedal flow in the right portal vein. Severely aliased flow is noted in two contiguous hepatic arteries. With the frequencies often used for color Doppler imaging (~3 MHz), flow within veins is often unaliased, while aliasing is common in arteries. Aliasing often enables differentiation of arteries and veins at a glance during real-time color Doppler scanning.

cent soft tissue (Figs. 29A and B). Artifact from tissue hum is generally greater in systole than in diastole.

In general, most of these artifacts can be recognized in the real-time examination once they are understood and have been seen a few times. If there is a question, spectral Doppler will generally, but not always, clarify the situation (Figs. 23A–D).

Ultrasound contrast agents promise to enhance the diag-

nostic abilities of sonographic imaging greatly. The use of ultrasound contrast agents, however, will probably add additional artifacts to color flow and spectral Doppler imaging. Color flow blooming may occur with the injection of contrast agents. Blooming is color overwritten on grayscale in regions where flow is not possible. In more subtle examples, blooming could overwrite areas of stenosis from clot or plaque, leading to false-negative results. Additionally, the use

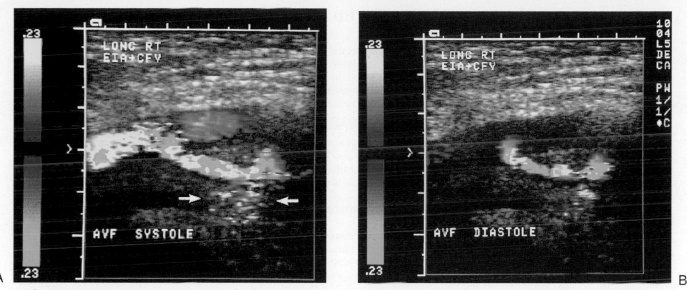

FIG. 29. Tissue hum: arteriovenous fistula. A: An arteriovenous fistula of the profunda femoris artery was caused by a stab wound. In systole, there is considerable tissue hum (*arrows*) adjacent to the pseudoaneurysm. B: This diastolic image reveals less tissue hum (tissue vibration). Blood flowing rapidly though the vascular abnormality causes tissue motion, displayed as color on the image.

of contrast agents may result in a 20% to 50% artifactual increase in the maximum spectral Doppler shifts detected. This may occur because of the limited dynamic range available on most ultrasound scanners; this could potentially result in actifactually high velocities. Another artifact is spectral bubble noise, which results in large excursions in the spectral and color display. Spectral bubble noise may be related to breakdown of microbubbles or the presence of very large individual bubbles in the contrast agent. Audibly, this sounds similar to a bubbling brook.

DESIRABLE QUALITIES FOR COLOR FLOW INSTRUMENTS

A color flow sonography system must have certain capabilities to generate good clinical color flow images. The greatest value of color flow imaging is that it enhances the overall diagnostic power of modern sonographic imaging. In survey color flow imaging, one scans a large area relatively quickly to detect areas of unsuspected flow or to differentiate vascular from nonvascular structures quickly. In this setting, system requirements include excellent sensitivity, a near-real-time frame rate, and adequate motion discrimination (the ability to differentiate blood flow from moving soft tissue). Sensitivity is important to detect unsuspected areas of flow easily. High frame rates are necessary to survey large areas quickly and to display the pulsatility of blood vessels and flow patterns within vessels. For example, high frame rates are helpful in differentiating among arteries and veins. Aliasing, which can make it impossible to determine flow direction, is tolerated in this "flow detection/survey" mode of scanning. Good motion discrimination, which enables the differentiation of moving red blood cells from moving soft tissue, is important to avoid artifacts that might obscure flow. Survey color flow imaging is most important in general scanning. Color Doppler is often preferable to power Doppler for survey purposes. Power Doppler, though more sensitive, is often too susceptible to motion artifacts for survey use.

Once an abnormality has been detected, the flow can be analyzed more closely—quality color flow imaging. In this situation, sensitivity and motion discrimination are again important. Aliasing is avoided by using an adequately high PRF. Resolution and registration are other key features. Registration is the accuracy with which a system displays the location of flow on the image. Resolution is the capability to depict small local variations in flow. This mode of color flow imaging is used initially in most vascular applications, since the location of the vessel to be evaluated is already known. Power Doppler flow imaging can provide added sensitivity in this setting. Of course, color flow can be used to guide placement of the spectral sample volume when detailed quantitative information is needed from a small area.

17

SUGGESTED READING

Burns PN. The physical principles of Doppler and spectral analysis. *J Clin Ultrasound* 1987;15:567–590.

Forsberg F, Liu JB, Burns PN, et al. Artifacts in ultrasonic contrast agent studies. *J Ultrasound Med* 1994; 13:357–365.

Kremkau FW. Doppler color imaging: principles and instrumentation. *Clin Diagn Ultrasound* 1992;27:7–60.

Merritt CRB. Doppler color flow imaging. *J Clin Ultrasound* 1987;15:591–597.

Middleton WD, Erickson SJ, Melson GL. Perivascular color artifact: pathologic significance and appearance on color Doppler ultrasound imaging. *Radiology* 1989;171:647–652.

Middleton WD, Melson GL. The carotid ghost: a color Doppler ultrasound duplication artifact. *J Ultrasound Med* 1990;9:487–491.

Mitchell DG. Color Doppler imaging: principles, limitations, and artifacts. *Radiology* 1990;177:1–10.

Nelson TR, Pretorius DH. The Doppler signal: where does it come from and what does it mean? *AJR* 1988; 151:439–447.

Pellerito JS, Troiano RN, Quedens-Case C, et al. Common pitfalls of endovaginal color Doppler flow imaging. *Radiographics* 1995;15:37–47.

Pozniak MA, Zagzebski JA, Scanlan KA. Spectral and color Doppler artifacts. *Radiographics* 1992;12:35–44.

Rubin JM, Bude RO, Carson PL, et al. Power Doppler ultrasound: potentially useful alternative to mean frequency based color Doppler ultrasound. *Radiology* 1994;190:853–856.

Rubin JM. AAPM tutorial: spectral Doppler. *Radiographics* 1994;14:139.

The Liver and Spleen

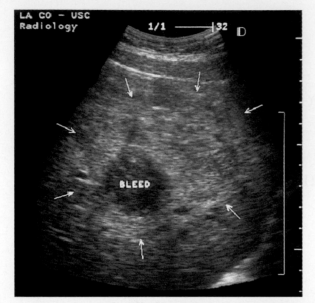

FIG. 30A. Grayscale.

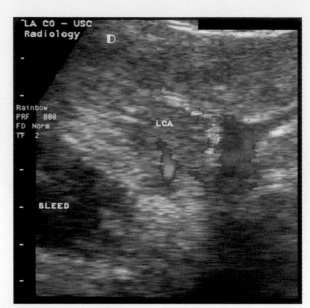

FIG. 30B. Color Doppler.

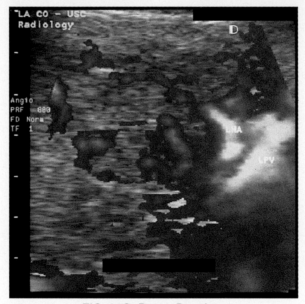

FIG. 30C. Power Doppler.

History

A 26-year-old female with acute, severe right upper-quadrant pain and mild hypotension.

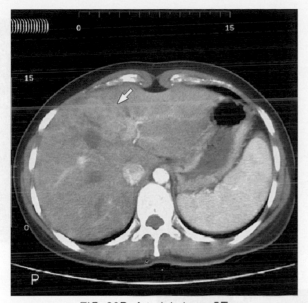

FIG. 30D. Arterial phase CT.

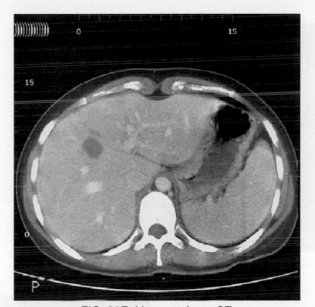

FIG. 30E. Venous phase CT.

Findings

Figure 30A is a transverse grayscale sonogram showing a large liver lesion that is slightly increased in echogenicity with some internal heterogeneity. A central, more hypoechoic portion is identified. Other areas of the liver were similarly abnormal. Figure 30B is a color Doppler sonogram that reveals flow around the periphery and a small amount of internal flow into this liver cell adenoma. Figure 30C, a power Doppler sonogram of the region of the adenoma, shows peripheral and internal flow. Note that the flow depiction is more robust than that seen in the color Doppler sonogram. Figure 30D is a double-spiral computed tomographic (CT) scan. On the arterial phase, the fairly intense enhancement in the adenoma to the right of the distal left portal vein (arrow) represents arterial enhancement of the liver cell adenoma. The ovoid lower-attenuation area within the dorsal portion of the mass is hemorrhage. The branching lower-attenuation areas more dorsally are unopacified hepatic veins. Figure 30E shows the venous phase CT, in which the adenoma is slightly less attenuating than the surrounding normal liver. The hematoma is highlighted to advantage by the enhancing hepatic parenchyma.

Diagnosis

Liver cell adenoma with acute hemorrhage.

Discussion

Liver cell adenoma has a variable pattern on grayscale and color Doppler, CT, and magnetic resonance imaging (MRI). Delayed imaging with hepatobiliary contrast agents, either with nuclear medicine techniques or MRI, may be useful. Because adenomas lack bile ducts, excretion of these agents is delayed, resulting in prolonged enhancement, generally not seen on early images. Hemorrhage into these lesions may be helpful in suggesting the diagnosis. After hemorrhage, identification of the actual adenoma may prove difficult. Power Doppler sonography and double-spiral CT in the arterial phase have the potential to enhance identification of liver cell adenomas. Treatment of liver cell adenomas has traditionally been surgical. With the advent of interventional radiologic techniques, more conservative management with therapeutic embolization may be appropriate in some cases.

Reference

Rummeny E, Saini S, Compton CC. Benign tumors of the liver. In: Freeny PC, Stevenson GW, eds. *Margolis and Burhenne's alimentary tract radiology*. St. Louis: CV Mosby, 1994:1645–1651.

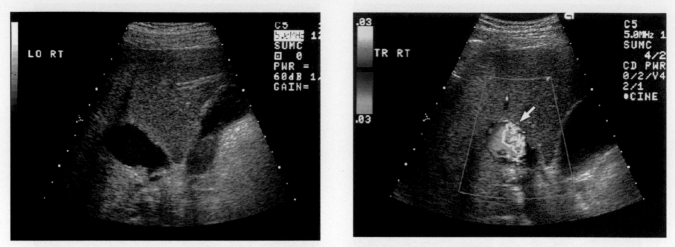

FIG. 31A. Grayscale.   FIG. 31B. Color Doppler.

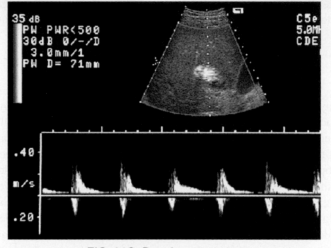

FIG. 31C. Doppler spectrum.

History

A 54-year-old male with fever and vague right upper-quadrant pain. Rule out liver abscess.

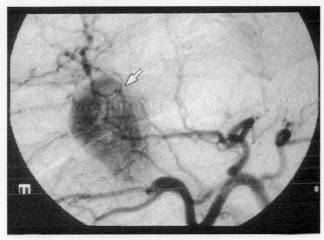

FIG. 31D. Arteriogram.

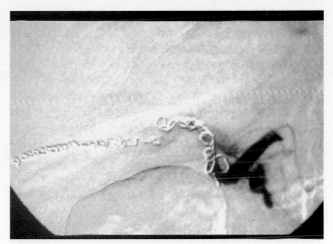

FIG. 31E. Arteriogram.

Findings

Figure 31A, a grayscale sagittal sonogram of the liver, demonstrates a cystic mass in the anterior segment of the right lobe. Note the color flow within the mass in Fig. 31B (arrow). A spectral Doppler tracing (Fig. 31C) demonstrates arterial flow consistent with an aneurysm. Figure 31D is an arteriogram demonstrating a large right hepatic artery mycotic aneurysm (arrow). This was selectively embolized (Fig. 31E).

Diagnosis

Mycotic aneurysm of the right hepatic artery secondary to endocarditis.

Discussion

Abdominal mycotic aneurysms are rare. The most common location is the supraceliac aorta. In many patients, a clear etiology is never found. Others, as in this case, ultimately prove to have bacterial endocarditis. Hepatic mycotic aneurysms may occur following liver transplantation. They may rupture and cause hemoperitoneum or hemobilia. Hepatic artery pseudoaneurysms are most commonly related to trauma or percutaneous interventions, such as biliary drainage procedures. One of the most important aspects of this case was evaluation of the cystic mass with color Doppler to diagnose the "cyst" correctly as a pseudoaneurysm. The diagnosis could easily have been missed with grayscale imaging alone. Because of low-volume flow within a pseudoaneurysm, pulsations often cannot be observed with real-time imaging alone. Thus, color Doppler is essential to the evaluation of all "cystic masses." This patient had a successful outcome following angiographic embolization and prolonged intravenous antibiotic therapy.

References

Khoda J, Lantsberg L, Sebbag G. Hepatic artery mycotic aneurysm as a cause of hemobilia [Letter]. *J Hepatol* 1993;17:131–132.

Rogers DW, Lumeng L, Goulet RJ, Canal DF. Ruptured mycotic pseudoaneurysm of the gastroduodenal artery presenting with hemoperitoneum and subcapsular liver hematoma. *Dig Dis Sci* 1990;35:661–664.

Sanchez-Bueno F, Robles R, Ramirez P, et al. Hepatic artery complications after liver transplantation. *Clin Transplant* 1994;8:399–404.

CASE 3

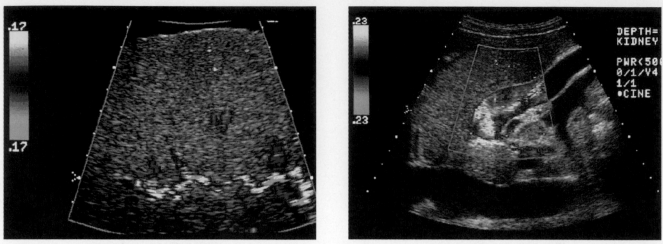

FIG. 32A. Color Doppler.

FIG. 32B. Color Doppler.

History

A 61-year-old cirrhotic male referred to sonography for evaluation for portosystemic collaterals.

Findings

Figure 32A is a transverse color Doppler sonogram through the right lobe of the liver. A small amount of ascites is seen adjacent to the ventral surface of the liver. The surface is nodular, compatible with a diagnosis of cirrhosis. The reversed flow (coded blue) in a small portal vein (arrow) represents hepatofugal portal flow, away from the periphery of the liver. An enlarged, tortuous hepatic artery runs horizontally through the figure. Flow is rapid, resulting in aliasing. Figure 32B is a longitudinal color Doppler sonogram of the region of the left portal vein. Note the hepatofugal flow via the large recanalized paraumbilical vein. The vein continues caudally in the ascitic fluid below the color box. For this reason, no flow is shown in this area.

Diagnosis

Color Doppler changes associated with portal hypertension and cirrhosis.

Discussion

Color flow sonography is a useful tool in evaluating patients with hepatic cirrhosis and its complications. In this patient, we see flow reversal and recanalization of the paraumbilical vein, both as a result of portal venous hypertension. Hepatofugal flow via a paraumbilical collateral is the second most common portosystemic collateral that occurs in portal hypertension. The most common is flow reversal in the coronary vein (also known as the left gastric vein). Flow reversal in the left gastric vein collateral results in esophageal varices. The enlarged and tortuous artery with rapidly flowing blood is another color flow sonographic finding sometimes seen in cirrhosis. This appearance is very similar to the angiographic "corkscrew artery" often seen in cirrhotic patients. Because of diminished or negative portal venous blood flow, patients with cirrhosis often have increased arterial flow, presumably as a homeostatic mechanism to maintain liver perfusion.

Reference

Ralls PW. Color Doppler sonography of the hepatic artery and portal venous system. *AJR* 1990;155:517–525.

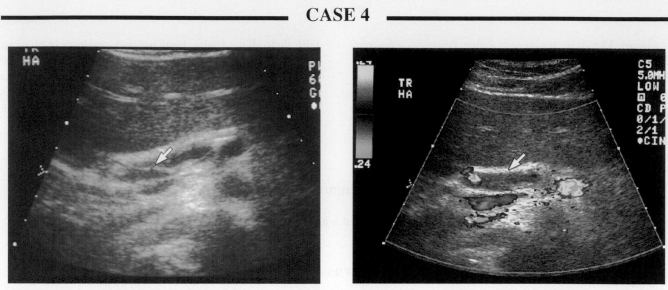

FIG. 33A. Grayscale.   FIG. 33B. Color Doppler.

History

A 32-year-old male with sudden onset of sharp right upper-quadrant pain and mild elevation of liver function test results. Rule out biliary colic.

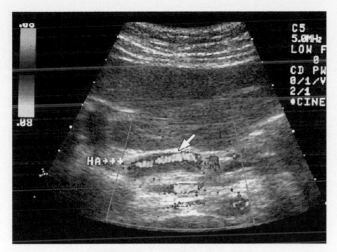

FIG. 33C. Color Doppler.

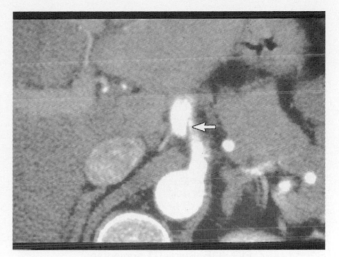

FIG. 33D. Spiral CT angiogram.

Findings

Figure 33A, a transverse sonogram of the celiac axis, demonstrates an intimal flap in the common hepatic artery (arrow). Figures 33B and C are color Doppler sonograms demonstrating a short segment occlusion of the proximal common hepatic artery. Note that Fig. 33C shows a patent distal true lumen (arrow), but thrombosis of the false lumen of the hepatic artery. Figures 33D–G are from a spiral CT angiogram. Figure 33D demonstrates an intimal flap (arrow) in the proximal celiac axis. Figure 33E is a curved planar reformation demonstrating a short segment occlusion of the common hepatic artery (arrow) and thrombosis of the distal false lumen. There is reconstitution of the distal hepatic artery via collaterals. Figure 33F is an axial scan demonstrating thrombosis of the false lumen adjacent to the patent distal right and left hepatic arteries. Figure 33G is a collapsed superior-to-inferior maximum-intensity projection view demonstrating the short segment occlusion of the common hepatic artery with collateral flow distally. Figures 33H and I are arteriograms. A celiac injection (Fig. 33H) demonstrates the short occlusion of the common hepatic artery with reconstitution of the distal hepatic artery via gastroduodenal collaterals from the superior mesenteric artery (Fig. 33I).

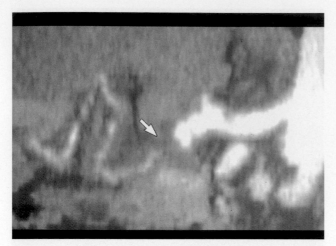

FIG. 33E. Spiral CT angiogram.

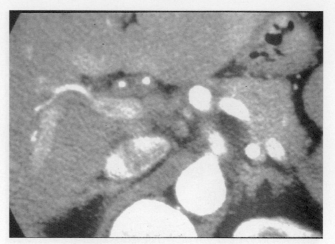

FIG. 33F. Spiral CT angiogram.

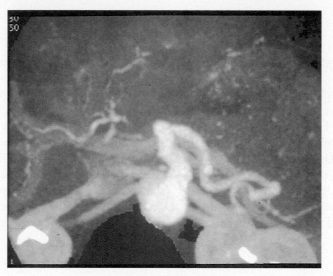

FIG. 33G. Spiral CT angiogram.

Diagnosis

Acute hepatic artery dissection due to Ehlers–Danlos syndrome.

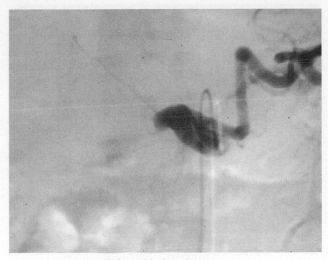

FIG. 33H. Arteriogram.

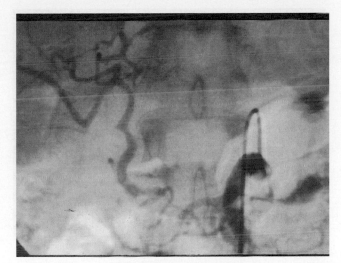

FIG. 33I. Arteriogram.

Discussion

The sudden episode of right upper-quadrant pain in this patient was caused by an acute hepatic artery dissection. This episode ultimately proved to be secondary to Ehlers–Danlos syndrome, type IV. These patients have defective collagen synthesis and are prone to aneurysm formation, intimal dissection, and vascular rupture. The imaging hallmark of a dissection is the identification of an intimal flap separating the true and false lumens. If Ehlers–Danlos syndrome is clinically suspected as the cause of an aneurysm or dissection, diagnostic angiography should be avoided because even minimal guidewire manipulation may cause arterial rupture. In this case, the patient's abdominal pain was clinically misdiagnosed as acute biliary colic. This underscores the need for a thorough vascular evaluation of the upper abdomen as a routine part of the sonographic study.

References

Mattar SG, Kumar AG, Lumsden AB. Vascular complications in Ehlers–Danlos syndrome. *Am Surg* 1994; 60:827–831.

Yoon DY, Park JH, Chung JW, Han JK, Han MC. Iatrogenic dissection of the celiac artery and its branches during transcatheter arterial embolization for hepatocellular carcinoma: outcome in 40 patients. *Cardiovasc Intervent Radiol* 1995;18:16–19.

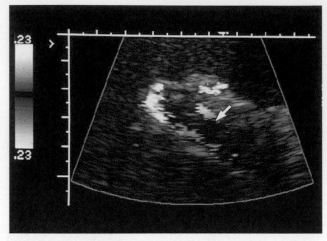

FIG. 34A. Color Doppler.

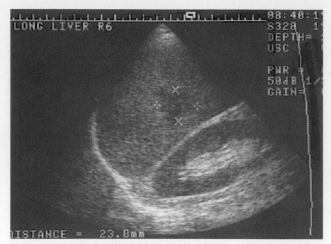

FIG. 34B. Grayscale.

History

A 50-year-old male who had an uneventful appendectomy for appendicitis, but returned 6 weeks later with recurrent fever and right upper-quadrant and lower-quadrant pain. Sonography was ordered to seek a cause for the pain.

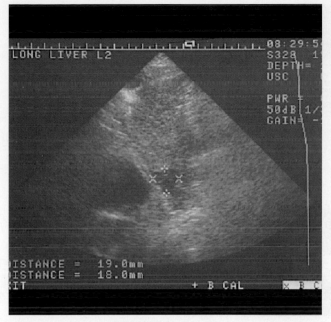

FIG. 34C. Grayscale.

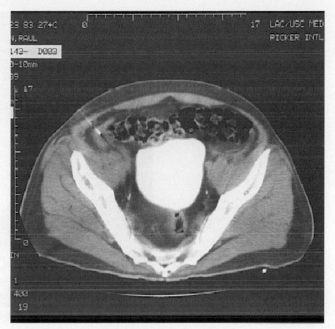

FIG. 34D. CT aspiration.

Findings

Figure 34A, a color Doppler sonogram through the right portal vein, revealed a substantial clot (arrow), indicative of pylephlebitis. Figure 34B, a longitudinal sonogram through the right lobe of the liver, revealed an ill-defined 3-cm lesion compatible with abscess. Figure 34C, a longitudinal grayscale image through the left lobe, revealed a 2-cm low-attenuation abscess in a juxtadiaphragmatic location. Figure 34D shows CT-guided aspiration of the right lower-quadrant fluid collection. A CT of the abdomen and pelvis was performed to seek out an intra-abdominal location as a presumed source for pylephlebitis with liver abscess. A right lower-quadrant fluid collection yielded pus on aspiration. Figure 34E shows the CT-guided percutaneous drainage of this abscess. The patient's fever quickly subsided on antibiotic treatment. Figure 34F, a color Doppler sonogram of the right portal vein 9 days later, reveals almost complete resolution of the previously noted right portal venous clot (arrow). Figure 34G, a repeat color Doppler sonogram of the right portal vein 5 weeks after Fig. 34F, reveals complete resolution of the portal venous clot.

31

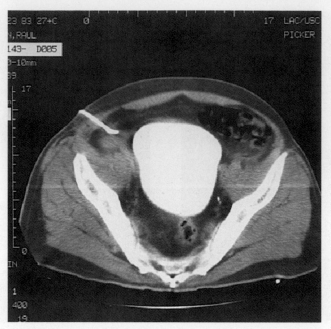

FIG. 34E. CT drainage.

Diagnosis

Pylephlebitis and liver abscess.

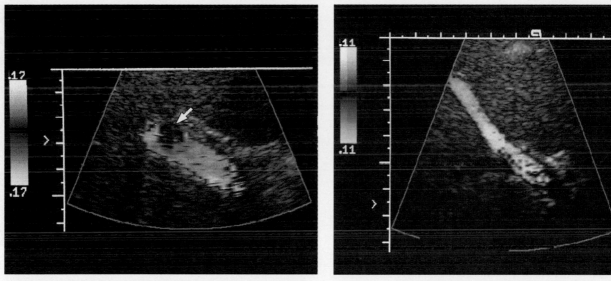

FIG. 34F. Color Doppler at 9 days.   FIG. 34G. Color Doppler at 6 weeks.

Discussion

Ascending infection by way of and involving the portal system is often called pylephlebitis, which is often accompanied by septic venous thrombosis. In this patient, pylephlebitis was a delayed complication of appendicitis. Color Doppler and grayscale sonography were used to identify the portal venous thrombus and the accompanying liver abscesses confidently. Liver abscess is a common complication of pylephlebitis. In these patients, the use of anticoagulants is unnecessary. The administration of antibiotics alone, as in this case, suffices to effect successful management. The prognosis for patients with liver abscesses associated with pylephlebitis is no worse than for patients with other liver abscesses. When appropriate, percutaneous drainage is effective in treating liver abscess. These smaller liver abscesses responded to antibiotics alone.

References

Jeffrey RB Jr, Ralls PW. The liver. In: *CT and sonography of the acute abdomen*. 2nd ed. Philadelphia: Lippincott–Raven, 1996:62–65.

Lim GM, Jeffrey RB Jr, Ralls PW, et al. Septic thrombosis of the portal vein: CT and clinical observations. *J Comput Assist Tomogr* 1989;13:656–658.

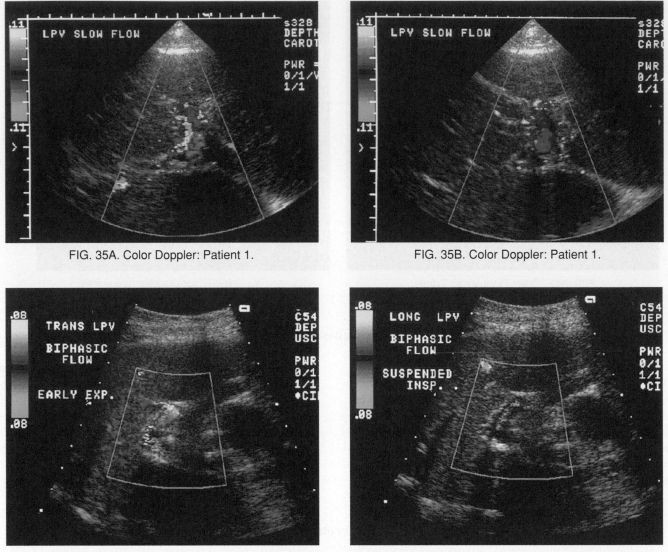

FIG. 35A. Color Doppler: Patient 1.

FIG. 35B. Color Doppler: Patient 1.

FIG. 35C. Color Doppler: Patient 2.

FIG. 35D. Color Doppler: Patient 2.

History

Two patients with portal hypertension.

Findings

Figure 35A, a color Doppler sonogram of the left portal vein, shows antegrade flow in the distal left portal vein (hepatopedal flow). Note the enlarged arteries that have aliased flow, especially the left hepatic artery that runs contiguously along the right side of the portal vein. Figure 35B shows flow reversal in the left portal vein in the same patient, in whom biphasic flow occurred with a pattern identical to the heart rate. Figure 35C, a transverse color Doppler sonogram of the left portal vein, reveals hepatopedal flow in early expiration. Figure 35D, a longitudinal sonogram of the left portal vein, reveals reversed flow (hepatofugal flow) during suspended inspiration.

Diagnosis

Two patients with biphasic portal flow; portal hypertension.

Discussion

Biphasic portal venous flow occurs in several conditions. One of the most striking of these is in patients with tricuspid regurgitation in whom alternate hepatopedal and hepatofugal flow occur with the beating heart. Biphasic flow can also be a feature of portal hypertension. In this circumstance, flow is generally slow. The "balance" of portal venous flow can be altered by physiologic influences. In Figs. 35A and B, the increased sinusoidal pressure during systole resulted in transient hepatofugal/reversed flow. In patient 2, the increased intra-abdominal pressure created by sustained inspiration increased sinusoidal pressures to the point where flow reversed. In most other phases of respiration, flow was hepatopedal in this patient.

Reference

Ralls PW. Color Doppler sonography of the hepatic artery and portal venous system. *AJR* 1990;155:517–525.

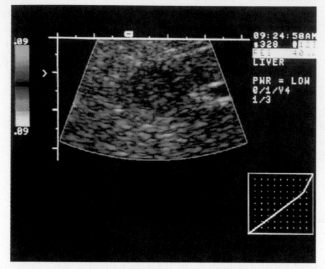

FIG. 36A. Color Doppler: Patient 1.

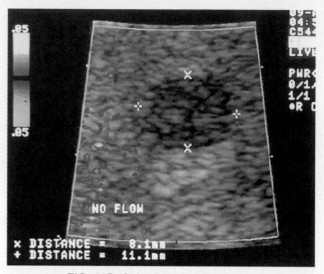

FIG. 36B. Color Doppler: Patient 2.

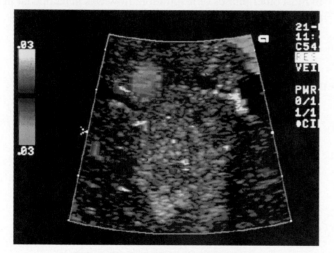

FIG. 36C. Color Doppler: Patient 3.

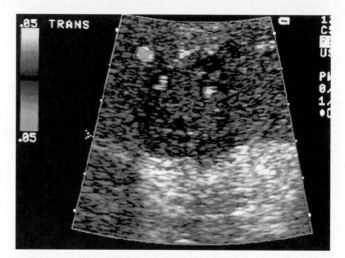

FIG. 36D. Color Doppler: Patient 4.

History

Six different patients.

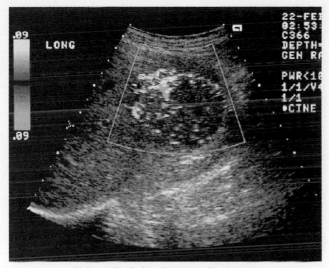

FIG. 36E. Color Doppler: Patient 5.

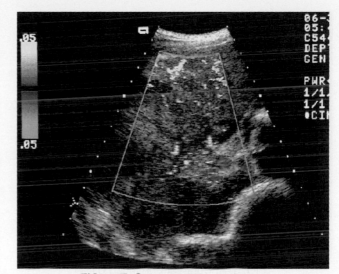

FIG. 36F. Color Doppler: Patient 6.

Findings

Figure 36A shows colon carcinoma liver metastasis with no internal or peripheral flow. Figure 36B shows pancreatic carcinoma liver metastasis with no internal or peripheral flow. Figure 36C demonstrates metastatic adenocarcinoma from an unknown primary with internal flow approximately equal to that of the liver in normal liver tissue. Figure 36D shows gastric carcinoma liver metastasis with slightly increased flow compared with the normal parenchyma. Figure 36E demonstrates renal cell carcinoma liver metastasis with markedly increased flow compared with normal liver parenchyma. Figure 36F shows pancreatic carcinoma liver metastasis with markedly increased flow compared with the normal liver.

Diagnosis

Color flow in hepatic metastasis.

Discussion

The majority of hepatic metastases (~66%) show no imageable color flow on color Doppler sonography. The remaining one-third have varying degrees of peripheral and internal color flow, as illustrated in Figs. 36C–F. Although detecting color flow in focal hepatic liver lesions should raise the index for suspicion for hepatocellular cancer (75% to 80% prevalence), flow also occurs frequently in hepatic metastasis (~33% prevalence). In fact, in the United States, any individual focal hepatic lesion that has internal flow is more likely to be metastasis than hepatocellular cancer, because metastases are so much more frequent than hepatocellular cancer (15 to 20 times greater prevalence in the United States).

References

Nino-Murcia M, Ralls PW, Jeffrey RB Jr, et al. Color flow Doppler characterization of focal hepatic lesions. *AJR* 1992;159:1195–1197.
Tanaka S, Kitamura T, Fujita M, et al. Color Doppler imaging of liver tumors. *AJR* 1990;154:509–514.

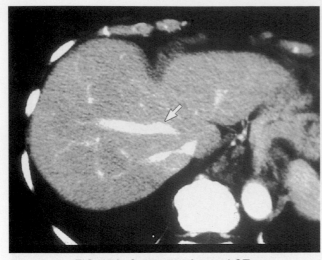

FIG. 37A. Contrast-enhanced CT.

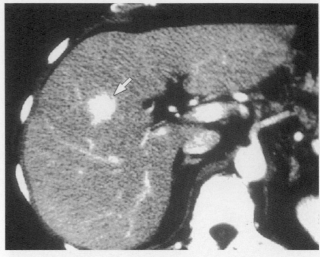

FIG. 37B. Contrast-enhanced CT.

History

A 61-year-old female with a hypervascular lesion noted on contrast-enhanced spiral CT of the liver. Rule out hepatic neoplasm.

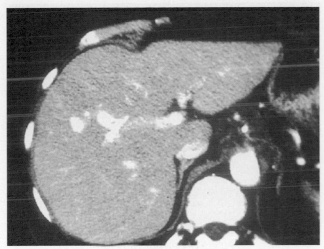

FIG. 37C. Contrast-enhanced CT.

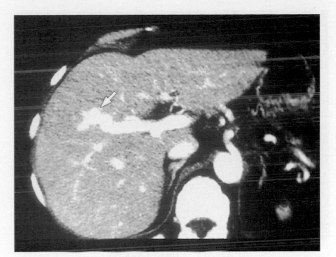

FIG. 37D. Contrast-enhanced CT.

Findings

Figures 37A–D are contrast-enhanced CT scans of the liver. Notice in Fig. 37A the relative enlargement of the middle hepatic vein (arrow) compared with the right and left hepatic veins. Figure 37B demonstrates contrast enhancement centrally within a high-attenuation lesion in the anterior segment of the right lobe (arrow). Figures 37C and D demonstrate direct communication between this enhancing area and the anterior division of the right portal vein (arrow, Fig. 37D). Figures 37E and F are power Doppler sonograms demonstrating a portal vein to hepatic vein communication (arrow, Fig. 37E). Note in Fig. 37G, which is a spectral Doppler tracing, the monophasic waveform of the middle hepatic vein due to the direct portal venous communication.

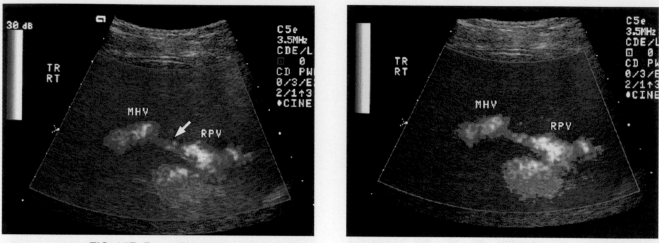

FIG. 37E. Power Doppler.   FIG. 37F. Power Doppler.

Diagnosis

Portal venous aneurysm secondary to hepatic vein to portal vein fistula.

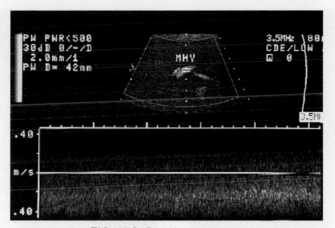

FIG. 37G. Doppler spectrum.

Discussion

This patient had a congenital portal vein to hepatic vein fistula. Over a long period, the turbulent flow within the fistula resulted in a venous aneurysm. Unlike the monophasic portal veins, with spectral Doppler analysis, the normal hepatic veins demonstrated a biphasic waveform due to the combination of antegrade flow and retrograde flow (from right atrial systole). Because of the direct communication to the portal vein, the bidirectional flow pattern was lost and the hepatic vein demonstrated a monophasic waveform. Space-occupying masses of the liver adjacent to the major hepatic veins can also "dampen" the hepatic venous waveform. The area of increased enhancement on the spiral CT could have been mistaken for an aneurysm or a hypervascular tumor. The color Doppler sonogram clearly identified this as a venous aneurysm related to the portal to hepatic vein fistula.

References

Gheorghu D, Liebowits O, Bloom RA. Case report: asymptomatic aneurysmal intrahepatic porto-hepatic venous shunt: diagnosis by ultrasound. *Clin Radiol* 1994;49:64–65.

Kudo M, Tomita S, Tochio H, Minowa K, Todo A. Intrahepatic portosystemic venous shunt: diagnosis by color Doppler imaging. *Am J Gastroenterol* 1993;88:723–729.

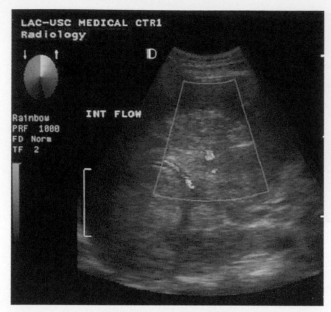

FIG. 38A. Color Doppler.

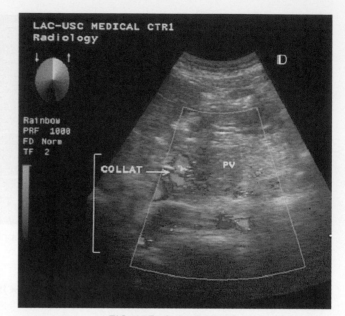

FIG. 38B. Color Doppler.

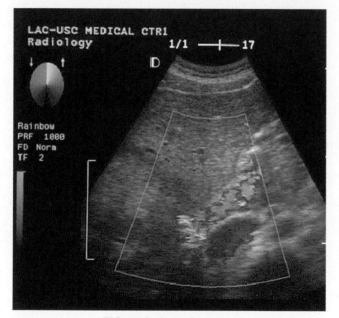

FIG. 38C. Color Doppler.

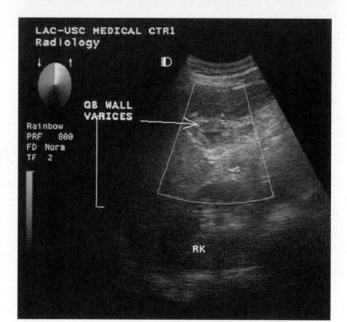

FIG. 38D. Color Doppler.

History

A 50-year-old male with right upper-quadrant pain and a 15-pound weight loss who had hepatitis B.

Findings

Figure 38A is a longitudinal oblique color Doppler sonogram through the right lobe of the liver. A large, mixed, primarily hyperechoic lesion is seen in the right lobe of the liver. Prominent internal flow and irregular vessels are noted within the mass. Multiple other masses were seen in other regions of the liver. Figure 38B, a transverse color Doppler sonogram through the hepatoduodenal ligament, demonstrates complete thrombosis of the portal vein. Contiguous collaterals are seen to the right of the thrombosed vessel. Figure 38C, a longitudinal color Doppler sonogram along the hepatoduodenal

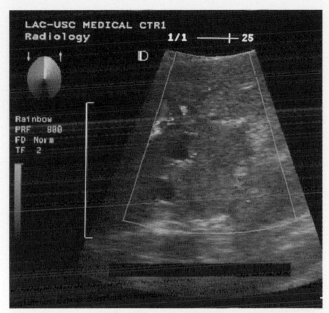

FIG. 38E. Color Doppler.

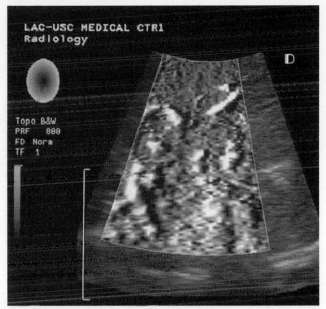

FIG. 38F. Power Doppler.

ligament, shows several hepatopedal collaterals within the ligament. Figure 38D, a transverse sonogram through the region of the gallbladder, shows several large portal venous collaterals within the gallbladder wall that are indicative of gallbladder varices. Figure 38E is a sagittal color Doppler sonogram showing complete thrombosis of the left portal vein and internal flow within the tumor thrombus. Small dilated ducts are noted cephalad to the tumor thrombus, as are slightly dilated arteries. Figure 38F, a power Doppler image of the left portal vein in the same location, demonstrates slightly more prominent flow within the tumor thrombus. This "topography" power Doppler flow map enhances the visualization of small vessels by displaying vascular edges more prominently.

Diagnosis

Sonographic complications of hepatocellular cancer.

Discussion

Hepatocellular carcinoma, which is the most common primary liver cancer, is much less common than hepatic metastases in the United States. Most hepatocellular carcinomas occur in patients with cirrhosis or precirrhotic conditions. Hepatitis-B-related cirrhosis has the highest prevalence of hepatocellular carcinoma, although hepatitis C may eventually be shown to be a more prevalent disease. In the United States, alcohol-related cirrhosis is the most common antecedent condition. Internal flow within hepatocellular carcinomas, as noted here, is usually seen in 75% of tumors in our experience. Venous invasion, especially portal venous invasion, is frequent. Involvement of the left and main portal veins, as noted here, reflects extensive disease. Flow within a thrombus is characteristic of neoplastic invasion rather than bland clot. Pulsatile spectral Doppler flow is virtually diagnostic of tumor. Rarely, a small amount of peripheral flow may be seen in veins filled with bland thrombus. Whenever the portal vein is completely occluded, as in this instance, hepatopedal collaterals may develop, which can result in cavernous transformation of the portal vein, a plexus of hepatopedal collaterals that bring blood to the liver, bypassing the occluded main portal vein. When veins in the gallbladder wall are recruited for collateral pathways for flow, gallbladder wall varices result, as in this instance. Color Doppler sonography is useful in showing the effects of hepatocellular carcinoma, as illustrated in this case.

References

Nino-Murcia M, Ralls PW, Jeffrey RB Jr, et al. Color flow Doppler characterization of focal hepatic lesions. *AJR* 1992;159:1195–1197.

Tanaka S, Kitamura T, Fugita M, Nakanishi K, et al. Color Doppler imaging in liver tumors. *AJR* 1990; 154:509–514.

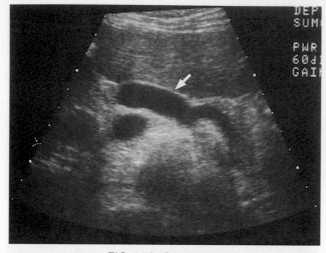

FIG. 39A. Grayscale.

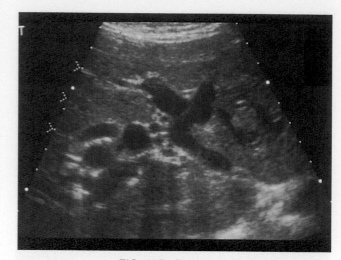

FIG. 39B. Grayscale.

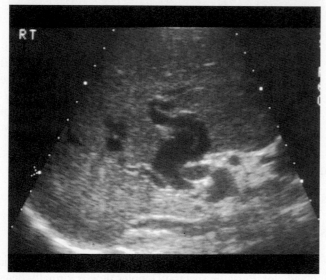

FIG. 39C. Grayscale.

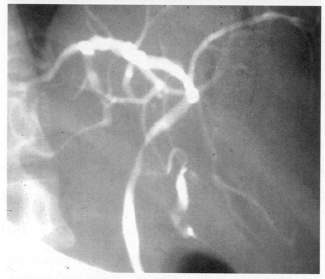

FIG. 39D. Endoscopic retrograde cholangiopancreatography.

History

A 54-year-old male with elevated liver function test results and whose outside sonogram was interpreted as demonstrating "dilated intrahepatic bile ducts."

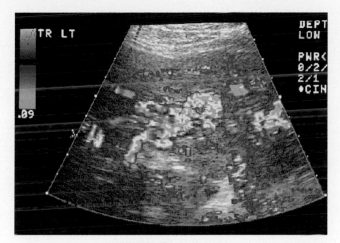

FIG. 39E. Color Doppler.

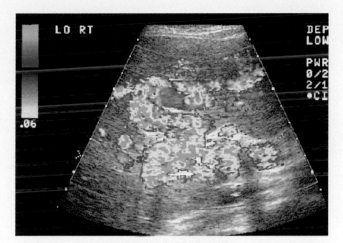

FIG. 39F. Color Doppler.

Findings

Figure 39A, a transverse grayscale image of the celiac axis, demonstrates marked enlargement of the diameter of the hepatic artery (arrow) compared with the splenic artery. Figure 39B, a transverse scan of the left lobe of the liver, shows dilated tubular structures throughout it. Figure 39C, a sagittal scan of the porta hepatis, demonstrates tortuous structures anterior to the portal vein. Figure 39D is an endoscopic retrograde cholangiopancreatography demonstrating extrinsic compression, but no dilatation of the intrahepatic bile ducts. Figures 39E and F are color Doppler sonograms of the liver that demonstrate marked hypervascularity of the liver with aliasing consistent with an arteriovenous malformation.

Diagnosis

Osler–Weber–Rendu disease with hepatic arteriovenous malformation.

Discussion

Osler–Weber–Rendu disease is the most common genetic cause of vascular bleeding. The liver is involved in up to 30% of patients. Although most often asymptomatic, either high-output congestive failure or gastrointestinal bleeding with hemobilia may rarely develop. In normal patients, the common hepatic and splenic arteries are approximately the same size. The marked enlargement of the hepatic artery in this case was caused by the dramatically increased flow from the hepatic arteriovenous malformation. This case underscores the value of the routine use of color Doppler in all cases of possible biliary obstruction. Because color Doppler sonography was not performed, the dilated intrahepatic vessels were at first mistakenly interpreted as dilated bile ducts on the outside sonogram. In selected patients, angiographic embolization may be of considerable value in reducing the hemodynamic effects of arteriovenous shunting.

References

Bourgeois N, Delcour C, Deviere J, et al. Osler–Weber–Rendu disease associated with hepatic involvement and high output heart failure. *J Clin Gastroenterol* 1990;12:236–238.

Ouchi K, Matsubara S, Mikuni J, Katayose Y, Endo K, Matsuno S. The radiologic presentation of Osler–Weber–Rendu disease of the liver. *Am J Gastroenterol* 1994;89:425–428.

Pompili M, Rapaccini GL, Marzano MA, et al. Doppler ultrasound findings in Osler–Weber–Rendu disease with hepatic involvement: a case report. *Ital J Gastroenterol* 1994;26:83–85.

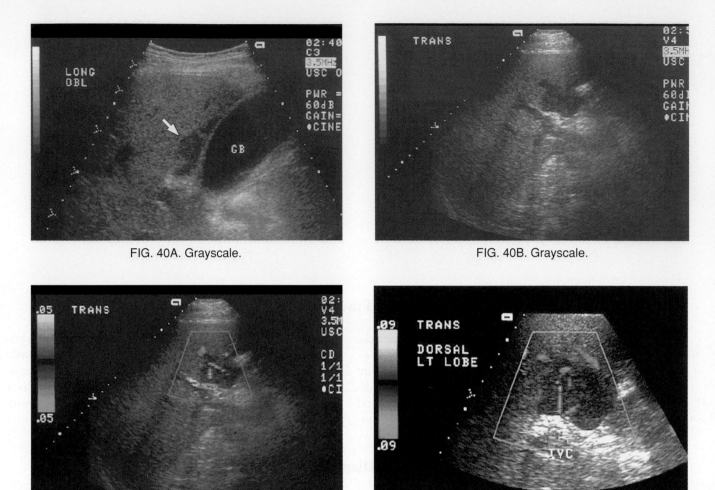

FIG. 40A. Grayscale.

FIG. 40B. Grayscale.

FIG. 40C. Color Doppler.

FIG. 40D. Color Doppler.

History

A 53-year-old male with right upper-quadrant pain and "dyspepsia" after eating. Right upper-quadrant sonography was requested.

Findings

Figure 40A, a longitudinal sonogram in the region of the gallbladder, revealed a lenticular area of decreased echogenicity (arrow) adjacent to the ventral surface of the gallbladder within the liver. This is a typical location and appearance for a spared area within a fatty liver. Increased hepatic echogenicity was also supportive of this diagnosis.

Figure 40B is a transverse sonogram through the same region, just cephalad to the gallbladder. Figure 40C, a color Doppler sonogram in the same location, reveals prominent internal flow within this hypoechoic area. Figure 40D, a magnified color Doppler sonogram of the same hypoechoic area, again reveals prominent internal flow.

Diagnosis

Prominent flow in a spared area within a fatty liver.

Discussion

Because of the unusual finding of increased flow within an apparently spared area within a fatty liver, a CT scan was requested. It revealed no abnormality whatever, other than fatty infiltration of the liver. No definite focal lesion was identified, nor was any evidence of increased enhancement in the region seen sonographically. With a biopsy performed under sonographic guidance, mild fatty infiltration of the liver was identified. Less affected regions within a fatty liver (so-called spared areas) may look like a conspicuous hypoechoic mass that simulates a neoplasm. The reason for this unusual apparent increased vascularity is uncertain. Generally, vessels run through both fatty areas and spared areas without being disturbed anatomically.

References

Caturelli E, Costarelli L, Giordano M, et al. Hypoechoic lesions in fatty liver. *Gastroenterology* 1991; 100:1678–1682.

White EM, Simeone JF, Mueller PR, et al. Focal periportal sparing in hepatic fatty infiltration: a cause of hepatic pseudomass on ultrasound. *Radiology* 1987;162:57 59.

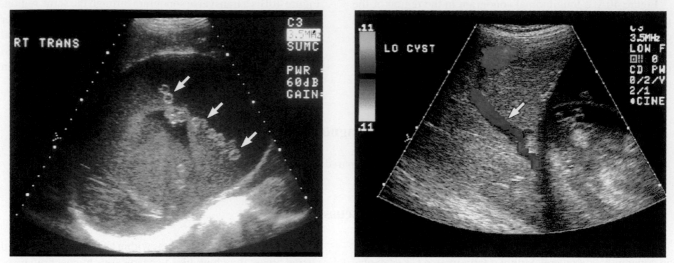

FIG. 41A. Grayscale.

FIG. 41B. Color Doppler.

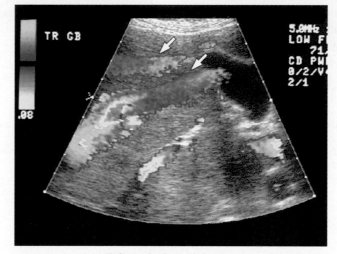

FIG. 41C. Color Doppler.

History

A 27-year-old female from Iran who had an enlarging right upper-quadrant mass and
vague abdominal pain.

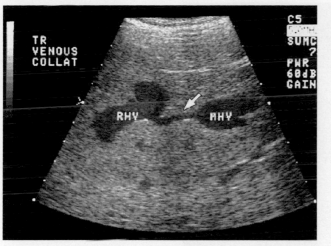

FIG. 41D. Grayscale.

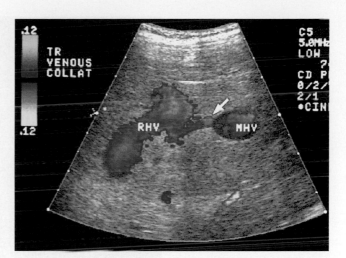

FIG. 41E. Color Doppler.

Findings

Figure 41A, a transverse scan of the right lobe of the liver, demonstrates a huge complex cystic mass obstructing the confluence of the hepatic veins. Note that within the mass are multiple rounded cystic structures (arrows). Figure 41B, a color Doppler sonogram of the right lobe of the liver, shows retrograde collateral (arrow) venous flow around the mass.

Figure 41C is another color Doppler sonogram demonstrating huge hepatic venous collaterals (arrows) flowing away from the liver. Figure 41D is a grayscale image showing communication (arrow) between the middle and right hepatic veins. This communication is clearly demonstrated with color Doppler imaging in Fig. 41E (arrow).

Diagnosis

Echinococcal cyst obstructing the hepatic venous confluence; hepatic vein to hepatic vein collaterals.

Discussion

Obstruction of the confluence of the hepatic veins in this patient undoubtedly occurred over a long period and resulted in extensive hepatic vein to hepatic vein collaterals. When obstruction of the hepatic venous confluence is present, pathways of venous drainage of the liver include diaphragmatic collaterals (phrenic veins) or retroperitoneal collaterals (azygous and lumbar veins). In this patient, the right hepatic venous system collateralized to the middle hepatic vein. Hepatic venous collaterals may be noted with color Doppler imaging in patients with Budd–Chiari syndrome and slow-growing hepatic tumors that obstruct the hepatic venous confluence. In Budd–Chiari

syndrome, the caudate lobe is relatively normal because of its direct venous communication to the inferior vena cava. Even though this patient had extensive hepatic venous collaterals, the results of her liver function tests were essentially normal, with only minimal elevation of alkaline phosphatase. This suggested that there was no underlying hepatic necrosis and that the collateral veins were essentially able to provide adequate venous outflow. Patients with Budd–Chiari syndrome, however, have histologic evidence of centrilobular congestion and necrosis.

References

Middleton MA, Middleton WD. Intrahepatic venous collaterals in a patient with congestive heart failure. *J Ultrasound Med* 1994;13:479–481.

Sakugawa H, Higashionna A, Oyakawa T, Kadena K, Kinjo F, Saito A. Ultrasound study in the diagnosis of primary Budd–Chiari syndrome (obstruction of the inferior vena cava). *Gastroenterol Jpn* 1992;27:69–77.

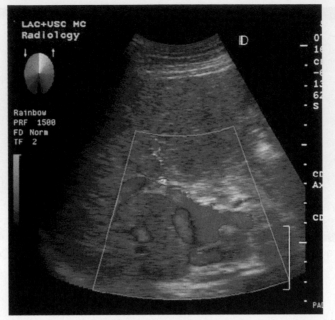

FIG. 42. Color Doppler.

History

A 32-year-old male referred to ultrasound because of right upper-quadrant pain.

Findings

Figure 42 is a transverse color Doppler sonogram showing dilatation of the right portal vein with swirling, red- and blue-coded flow. This is virtually diagnostic of a portal venous aneurysm. No other abnormalities were detected.

Diagnosis

Portal vein aneurysm.

Discussion

Portal venous aneurysms are rare vascular malformations that are considered congenital in etiology. They may be saccular or fusiform and range in size from 3 to 8 cm. Clinical sequelae are uncommon. Extrinsic compression of the duodenum, common bile duct, portal hypertension, venous thrombosis, and, rarely, rupture have been reported.

Reference

Cho KJ. Vascular diseases of the liver. In: Freeny PC, Stevenson GW, eds. *Margolis & Burhenne's alimentary tract radiology*. St. Louis: CV Mosby, 1994:1623.

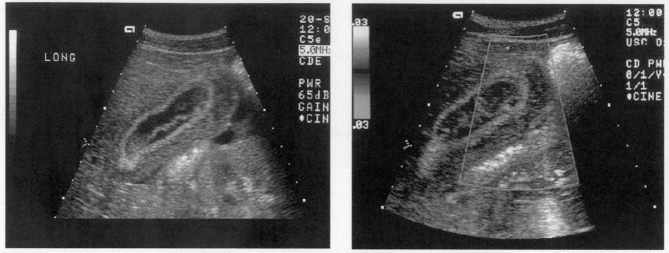

FIG. 43A. Grayscale.

FIG. 43B. Color Doppler.

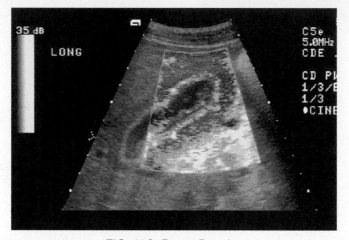

FIG. 43C. Power Doppler.

History

A 32-year-old male with mild jaundice, fever, and right upper-quadrant pain. Ultrasound was requested to rule out acute cholecystitis.

Findings

Figure 43A, a longitudinal sonogram of the gallbladder, reveals marked symmetric thickening of the gallbladder wall. Small striations are present, and an intraluminal linear echo, suggestive of an intraluminal membrane, is identified. Figure 43B, a color flow sonogram through the fundus of the gallbladder, shows flow near the submucosa. Figure 43C is a power Doppler sonogram showing diffuse submucosal and fundal flow. No gallstones were identified in the gallbladder.

Diagnosis

Hepatitis A, which mimics acute cholecystitis.

Discussion

This patient exhibited findings seen commonly in patients with hepatitis A. The absence of gallstones and the symmetric thickening of the gallbladder wall, coupled with laboratory findings of markedly elevated alanine aminotransferase and aspartate aminotransferase levels, made the diagnosis clear. Some of the most abnormal-appearing gallbladder walls occur in patients with hepatitis A. Potentially problematic findings occurred in this patient, however. The apparent intraluminal membrane, the marked gallbladder wall thickening with intramural striations, and the fundal and submucosal flow all have been described in gangrenous and severe acute cholecystitis. The nonspecificity of these findings is made clear by this case. Gallbladder wall thickening is a nonspecific finding that, although seen notably in hepatitis A, may occur in many conditions, including—but not limited to—HIV infection, hypoalbuminemia (especially when coupled with portal hypertension), and acute or chronic calculous cholecystitis. Sloughed mucosa, another sign of severe cholecystitis, may be simulated by intraluminal sludge, as in this case.

References

Ralls PW, Quinn MF, Jutner HU, et al. Gallbladder wall thickening: patients without intrinsic gallbladder disease. *AJR* 1991;137:65–68.

Teefey SA, Baron RL, Bigler SA. Sonography of the gallbladder: significance of striated (layered) thickening of the gallbladder wall. *AJR* 1991;156:945–947.

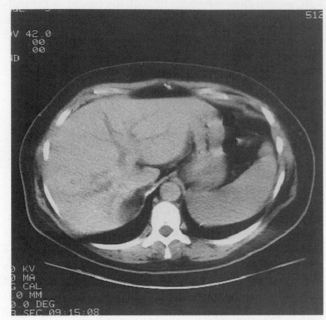

FIG. 44A. Contrast-enhanced CT.

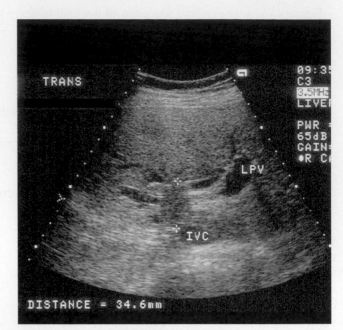

FIG. 44B. Grayscale.

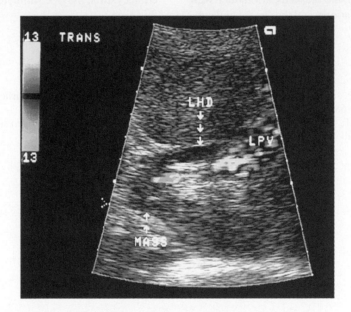

FIG. 44C. Color Doppler.

History

A 50-year-old female with jaundice and a 15-pound weight loss who had no pain or other complaints.

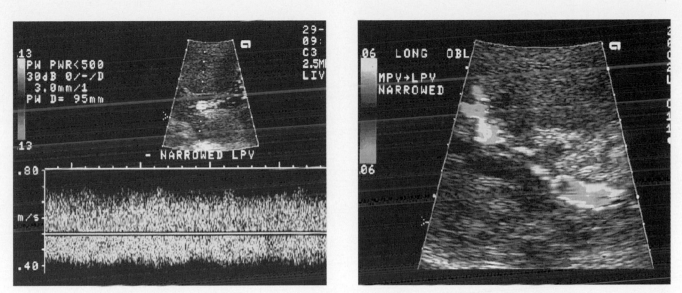

FIG. 44D. Doppler spectrum.   FIG. 44E. Color Doppler.

Findings

Figure 44A is poor-quality contrast-enhanced CT through the region of the left portal vein. This suboptimal CT shows biliary dilatation and some atrophy of the right lobe, but no discrete mass. The patient was referred for color Doppler sonographic evaluation of potential resectability. Figure 44B, a transverse grayscale sonogram through the region of the porta hepatis, reveals a cylindrically shaped mass that measures 3.5 cm in long axis. Dilatation of both left-sided and right-sided ducts is noted. Figure 44C, a transverse color Doppler sonogram in the region of the left portal vein, shows obstruction of a left-sided bile duct just ventral to the proximal portion of the left portal vein. The slight biliary ductal wall thickening suggests extension of tumor submucosally along this duct. Also noted is prominent narrowing of the proximal portion of the left portal vein. The more distal portal vein (labeled LPV) is of more normal caliber. Figure 44D, a spectral Doppler in the region of the narrow left portal vein, reveals turbulent high-velocity flow. Figure 44E is a longitudinal oblique color Doppler sonogram through the region of the distal main portal vein and proximal left portal vein. The mass narrows the proximal left portal vein. This confirms the findings on the lateral view (Fig. 44C).

Diagnosis

Unresectable cholangiocarcinoma. Color Doppler was used to evaluate resectability.

Discussion

Involvement of the right-sided second-order ducts (peripheral to the main right hepatic duct) plus the narrowed left portal vein mean that, because of bilateral disease, this patient cannot be treated by resection. At surgery, all of the sonographic findings were confirmed, including the extension of tumor into the left hepatic ducts (Fig. 44C). Criteria for unresectability, as demonstrated by color flow sonography, include main portal vein occlusion, left and right portal vein involvement, and extensive unilateral ductal obstruction of the second-order branch ducts with contralateral atrophy or vascular involvement. Evidence of disseminated disease including hepatic nodal and other metastases is also an indicator of unresectability. Recently, sonography has been shown to be as useful as angiography or arterial portography in determining resectability of malignant hilar cholangiocarcinomas.

References

Hann LE, Fong Y, Shriver CD, et al. Malignant hepatic hilar tumors: can ultrasonography be used as an alternative to angiography with CT arterial portography for determination of resectability? *J Ultrasound Med* 1996;15:37–45.
Stain SC, Baer HU, Dennison AR, et al. Current management of hilar cholangiocarcinoma. *Surg Gynecol Obstet* 1992;175:579–588.

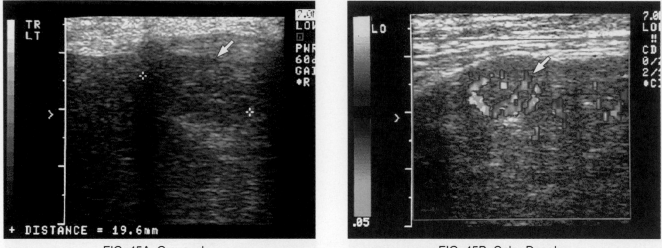

FIG. 45A. Grayscale.

FIG. 45B. Color Doppler.

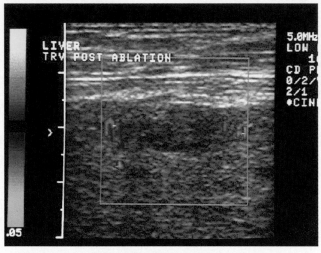

FIG. 45C. Color Doppler.

History

A 60-year-old male with elevated α-fetoprotein and normal abdominal CT and MRI findings. A sonogram at another hospital demonstrated no abnormality.

Findings

Figure 45A is a grayscale image of the surface of the liver with a high-resolution linear array transducer. Note the subtle hypoechoic mass (arrow, Fig. 45A), which is hypervascular on color Doppler (arrow, Fig. 45B). Biopsy performed using sonographic guidance was consistent with hepatocellular carcinoma. The tumor was treated with percutaneous alcohol ablation, again guided by sonography. A follow-up color Doppler sonogram (Fig. 45C) demonstrates no further vascularity within the mass, consistent with a good response to intramural injection of alcohol.

Diagnosis

Superficial hepatocellular carcinoma treated with alcohol ablation.

Discussion

Because of the standard focal zone of most abdominal transducers (3.5 to 5.0 MHz), small hepatic tumors within 1 cm of the liver capsule often go undetected. It is, therefore, essential to perform a dedicated survey of the surface of the liver by using a high-resolution (7.5 MHz) transducer. Color Doppler sonography was very helpful in this case in demonstrating the hypervascularity of the small hepatocellular carcinoma. The vascularity can also be used to guide and monitor the effects of alcohol ablation as the tumor vascularity markedly diminishes following injection of alcohol. Ethanol ablation has been quite successful in treating small (<3 cm) hepatocellular carcinomas. Multiple injections are usually required.

References

Lencioni R, Caramelia D, Bartolozzi C. Hepatocellular carcinoma: use of color Doppler US to evaluate response to treatment with percutaneous ethanol injection. *Radiology* 1995;194:113–118.

Nino-Murcia M, Ralls PW, Jeffrey RB Jr, Johnson M. Color flow Doppler characterization of focal hepatic lesions. *AJR* 1992;159:1195–1197.

Numata K, Tanaka K, Mitsui K, Morimoto M, Inoue S, Yonezawa H. Flow characteristics of hepatic tumors at color Doppler sonography: correlation with arteriographic findings. *AJR* 1993;160:515–521.

Yasuhara K, Kimura K, Nakamura H, Iwadare M, Ohto M, Matsuzaki O. Doppler velocity histogram analysis of hepatocellular carcinoma. *J Clin Ultrasound* 1995;23:225–231.

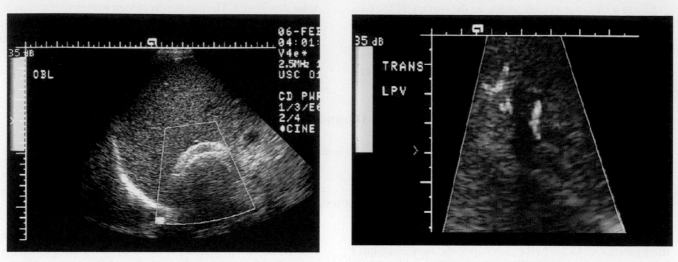

FIG. 46A. Color Doppler.
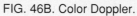
FIG. 46B. Color Doppler.

History

A 39-year-old male with alcoholic cirrhosis and variceal gastrointestinal bleeding who had a transjugular intrahepatic portosystemic shunt (TIPS) performed to decompress his portal venous hypertension and who, 2 weeks later, returned again with upper gastrointestinal bleeding. Color flow sonography was requested.

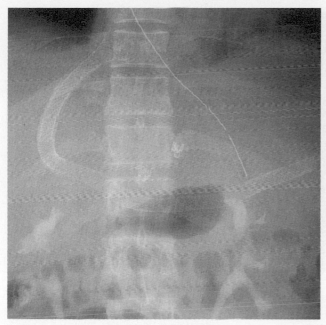

FIG. 46C. Radiograph.

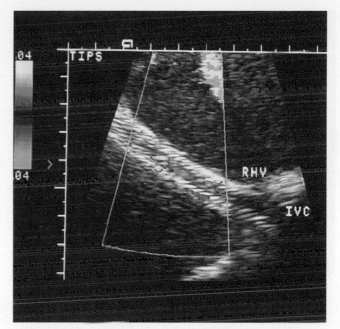

FIG. 46D. Color Doppler.

Findings

Figure 46A is a color Doppler sonogram revealing no flow within the TIPS stent, suggesting complete thrombosis. Figure 46B is a transverse color Doppler sonogram of the left portal vein with contiguous prominent arteries. Further evaluation revealed thrombosis of the entire portal venous system. The patient was taken to the interventional suite to reestablish patency of the stent. Figure 46C is an abdominal film revealing extension and recanalization of the previously placed TIPS stent. Five additional wall stents were placed through the clotted portal vein, confluence, and splenic vein. Figure 46D, color Doppler sonography subsequent to place-ment of the multiple stents to recanalize the portal venous system, reveals poor or absent flow within the intrahepatic stent. Figure 46E, a power Doppler sonogram of the intrahepatic TIPS stent, reveals flow throughout the stent, documenting patency. Power Doppler, with its enhanced sensitivity, shows flow throughout the entire system. Figure 46F is a power Doppler sonogram showing the patent stent reaching into the intrasplenic splenic vein. Figure 46G, a transverse sonogram of the spleen, shows the TIPS wall stent extending into the intraparenchymal splenic vein. This corresponds to the power Doppler image shown in Fig. 46F.

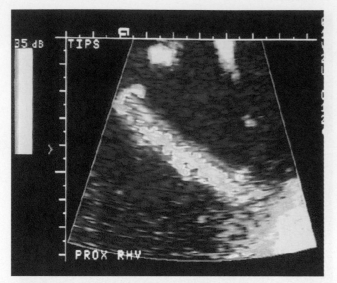

FIG. 46E. Power Doppler.

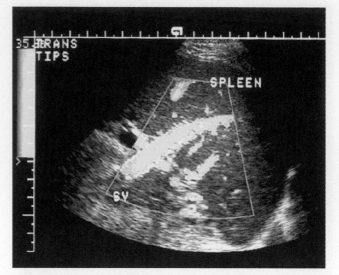

FIG. 46F. Power Doppler.

Diagnosis

Power Doppler visualization of a TIPS shunt.

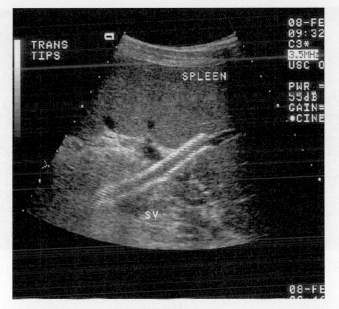

FIG. 46G. Grayscale.

Discussion

Unfortunately, many patients with TIPS stents are difficult to scan. Low frequency, low angle, and power Doppler are often necessary to demonstrate flow within TIPS stents, especially in difficult patients. The use of power Doppler enabled documentation of patency after this extensive restenting procedure.

References

Chong WK, Malisch TW, Mazer MJ, et al. Sonography of transjugular intrahepatic portiosystemic shunts. *Semin Ultrasound CT MR* 1995;16:69–80.
Foshagger MC, Ferral H, Nazarian GH, et al. Duplex sonography after TIPS: normal hemodynamic findings and efficacy in depicting shunt patency and stenosis. *AJR* 1995;165:1–7.

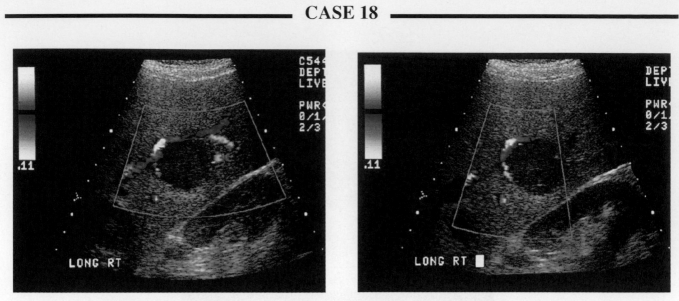

FIG. 47A. Color Doppler.   FIG. 47B. Color Doppler.

History

A 50-year-old male with known carcinoma of the lung and elevated liver function test results. Rule out liver metastasis.

Findings

Figures 47A and B are sagittal color Doppler sonograms of the right lobe of the liver. Note the hypoechoic solid lesion, which contains no intrinsic vascularity, but displaces adjacent hepatic vessels.

Diagnosis

Hepatic metastasis from carcinoma of the lung demonstrating the "detour" sign.

Discussion

Tanaka et al. described different color flow patterns for primary and metastatic hepatic neoplasms. Primary hepatic lesions such as hepatocellular carcinoma and focal nodular hyperplasia typically demonstrate intrinsic vascularity with a central or "basketlike" configuration. In addition to the central vascularity, hepatocellular carcinomas may demonstrate high-velocity flow from arteriovenous shunting. This finding is rarely, if ever, seen with metastatic disease. Hepatic metastases, on the other hand, are characterized by a peripheral displacement of vessels known as the "detour" sign. A more recent study by Nino-Murcia et al. suggests that there is significant overlap between these two patterns and that up to 25% of hepatocellular carcinomas do not demonstrate intrinsic vascularity and may mimic metastasis. Thus, for any given lesion, guided biopsy remains essential for accurate diagnosis.

References

Nino-Murcia M, Ralls PW, Jeffrey RB Jr, et al. Color flow Doppler characterization of focal hepatic lesions. *AJR* 1992;159:1195–1197.

Tanaka S, Kitamura T, Fujita M, et al. Color flow Doppler imaging of liver tumors. *AJR* 1990;154:509–514.

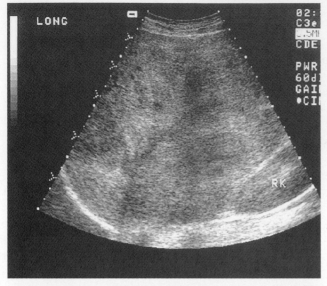

FIG. 48A. Grayscale.

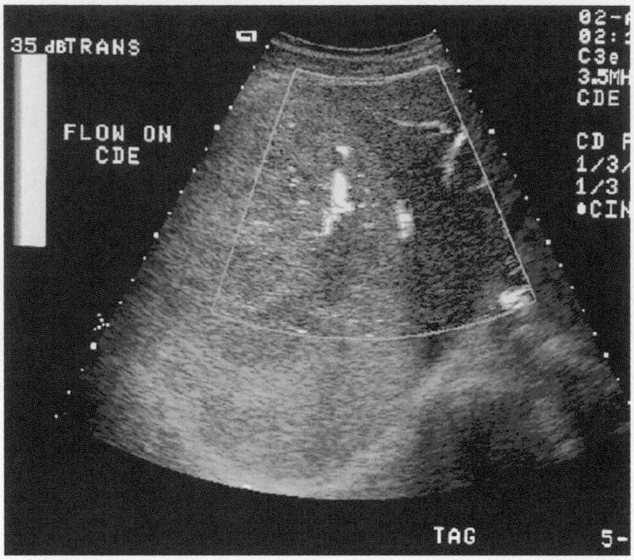

FIG. 48B. Power Doppler.

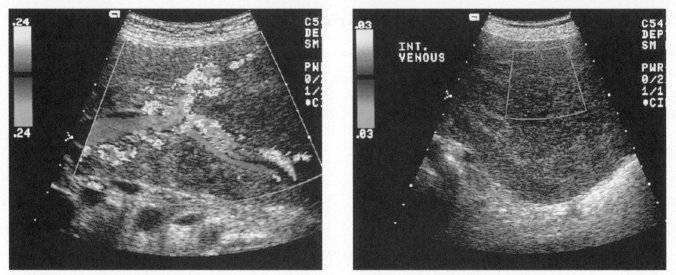

FIG. 48C. Color Doppler.

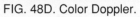

FIG. 48D. Color Doppler.

History

Most hemangiomas in the liver have flow that is too slow to be imaged sonographically. Large hemangiomas usually have imageable internal flow and often have unusual hemodynamics at the periphery of the lesion.

Findings

Figure 48A is a longitudinal sonogram of a large hemangioma, a lesion that measured 20 cm in long axis and had no feature that enabled a confident diagnosis of hemangioma. Figure 48B, a power Doppler sonogram obtained transversely through the boundary between the hemangioma and normal liver, reveals as much flow in the large hemangioma as is seen in the hepatic parenchyma. Figure 48C shows a second atypical hemangioma in the lateral segment of the left lobe of the liver. This huge hemangioma exhibits a small amount of internal venous flow. Despite low flow within the lesion itself, Fig. 48D, a transverse color Doppler sonogram in the region of the left portal vein, shows rapid and massive aberrant blood flow around the hemangioma. Multiple enlarged peripheral feeding arteries with aliased flow are noted. Blood draining from the hemangioma exits via the left portal vein and its branches. The surprising and rare finding of portal vein flow reversal is noted.

Diagnosis

Large hemangiomas of the liver: unusual color flow image findings.

Discussion

Cavernous hemangiomas of the liver are characterized by slow internal flow with large, slow flow vascular structures at the periphery. Imaging flow within hemangiomas with color flow sonographic imaging techniques may be difficult because of the slow velocities involved. Slowly flowing blood does not generate Doppler frequency shifts that are great enough to be readily detectable. Larger hemangiomas have a higher prevalence of internal flow than do smaller hemangiomas. Our experience suggests that the majority of large hemangiomas (>5 cm) have imageable internal flow on color Doppler. Imageable flow is much less common (<10%) in lesions under that size. The second case demonstrates flow reversal with drainage of blood via the portal system. The etiology of this is uncertain, but may be related to shunting within the hemangioma, or overloading the capacity of the hepatic venous system draining the left lobe because of the large amount of blood flowing through the lesion.

Reference

Nino-Murcia M, Ralls PW, Jeffrey RB Jr, et al. Color flow Doppler characterization of focal hepatic lesions. *AJR* 1992;159:1195–1197.

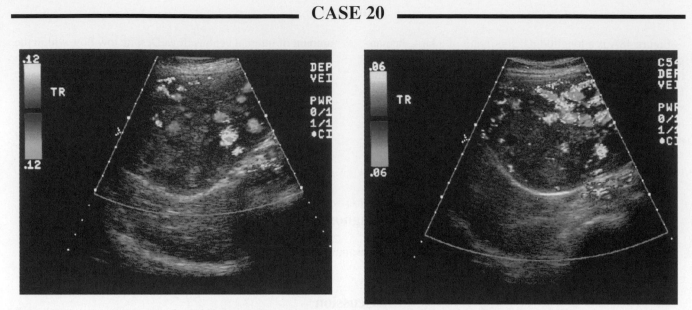

FIG. 49A. Color Doppler.   FIG. 49B. Color Doppler.

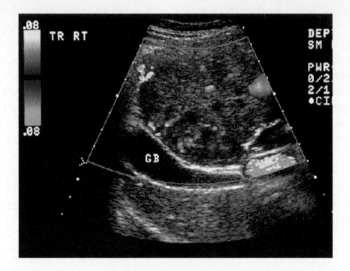

FIG. 49C. Color Doppler.

History

A 54-year-old female with known hepatitis C and increasing abdominal pain.

Findings

Figures 49A–C are transverse scans of the right lobe of the liver that demonstrate a predominantly hypoechoic mass containing prominent intrinsic vascularity.

Diagnosis

Hepatocellular carcinoma.

Discussion

Hepatocellular carcinoma is characterized by the presence of high-velocity Doppler signals representing arteriovenous shunting and intrinsic color Doppler flow within the lesion. The differential diagnosis includes hypervascular metastatic lesions (i.e., melanoma, islet cell carcinoma, and renal cell carcinoma). Focal nodular hyperplasia and hepatic adenomas are benign lesions that may also demonstrate intrinsic vascularity with color Doppler, but no evidence of arteriovenous shunting. Color Doppler imaging may aid in the ultrasound-guided biopsy of hypervascular lesions such as hepatocellular carcinoma. Large arteries within the lesion can clearly be identified and avoided during needle insertion.

References

Learch TJ, Ralls PW, Johnson MB, et al. Hepatic focal nodular hyperplasia: findings with color Doppler sonography. *J Ultrasound Med* 1993;12:541–544.

Nino-Murcia M, Ralls PW, Jeffrey RB Jr, et al. Color flow Doppler characterization of focal hepatic lesions. *AJR* 1992;159:1195–1197.

Tanaka S, Kitamura T, Fujita M, Nakanishi K, et al. Color flow Doppler imaging of liver tumors. *AJR* 1990; 154:509–514.

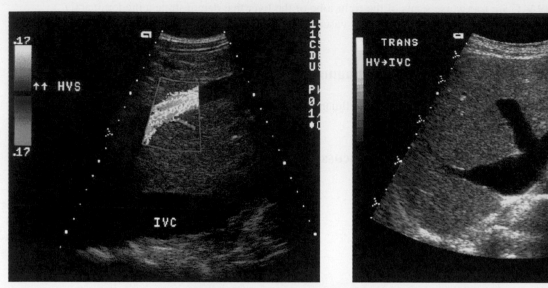

FIG. 50A. Color Doppler.

FIG. 50B. Grayscale.

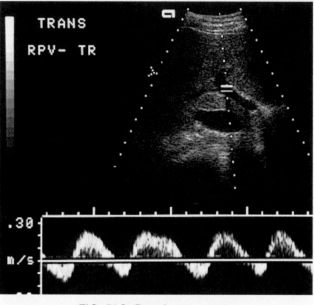

FIG. 50C. Doppler spectrum.

History

A 55-year-old male with a history of cardiac disease who had vague upper abdominal pain and abnormal liver function test results. Sonography was ordered.

Findings

Figure 50A, a longitudinal image of the liver, shows a markedly enlarged middle hepatic vein. Note the small tributary to the hepatic vein. Small hepatic venous tributaries are only occasionally imaged in normals. Figure 50B is a transverse sonogram showing the hepatic veins emptying into the inferior vena cava. The hepatic veins and inferior vena cava are larger than usual. Figure 50C, a transverse spectral Doppler sonogram of the right portal vein, reveals a biphasic portal venous waveform. Usually, the spectral waveform in the portal vein is monophasic with slight cardiac variations.

Diagnosis

Tricuspid insufficiency with enlarged hepatic veins and biphasic portal venous waveform.

Discussion

Tricuspid insufficiency, from intrinsic valvular disease or functional enlargement of the tricuspid valve orifice because of cardiac failure, causes increased right-sided pressures. The abnormal biphasic portal venous waveform noted in Fig. 50C is characteristic of tricuspid insufficiency. The phasic waveform observed is presumably related to transmission of increased right-sided pressures into the portal vein via the hep atic sinusoids. This portal vein waveform should suggest the possibility of tricuspid regurgitation. On occasion, other conditions that may result in similar waveforms include cirrhosis and constrictive pericarditis and may even be seen in well-conditioned athletes. Chronic elevation of right-sided pressures may eventually lead to hepatic cirrhosis due to chronic passive congestion.

Reference

Jeffrey RB Jr, Ralls PW. The liver. In: *Sonography of the abdomen.* Philadelphia. Lippincott–Raven, 1995:151.

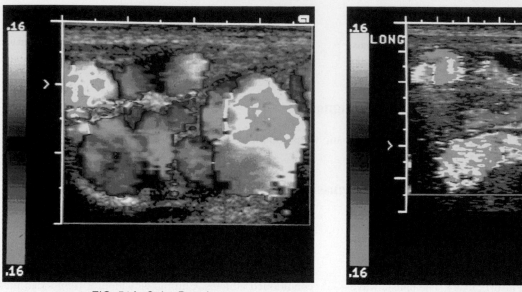

FIG. 51A. Color Doppler.   FIG. 51B. Color Doppler.

History

A 45-year-old female with chronic hepatitis B infection who was referred to ultrasound because of right upper-quadrant pain.

Findings

Figure 51A is a high-resolution color Doppler revealing tangles of superficial abdominal collaterals in the region between the xiphoid process and umbilicus. These collaterals arise from a recanalized paraumbilical vein (not shown). Figure 51B, a high-resolution color Doppler scan in the region of the umbilicus, reveals tortuous collaterals ramifying near and radiating from that region. This is the ultrasound equivalent of the physical findings of caput medusae. Multiple collaterals related to portosystemic shunting are seen in the area of the umbilicus.

Diagnosis

Portosystemic collaterals; paraumbilical sonographic caput medusae.

Discussion

Recanalization of paraumbilical veins is the second most common portosystemic collateral that occurs in association with hepatic cirrhosis. The most common is flow reversal in the left gastric (coronary) vein. Paraumbilical collaterals usually communicate with superficial abdominal collaterals, as in this case. These collaterals frequently ramify in the region of the umbilicus, forming a color Doppler "caput medusae" appearance. Color Doppler sonography is more sensitive in detecting these paraumbilical collaterals. Often, these tortuous collaterals cannot be identified by visual inspection—they may not result in the classic physical examination pattern of findings. Collaterals from this location may communicate with the femoral venous circulation via the inferior epigastric vein or may descend into the pelvis, communicating with the iliac veins or even the perirectal venous plexus. When this last occurs, dilated hemorrhoidal veins may result. These findings have little clinical significance. Identifying these paraumbilical collaterals may be important before laparoscopy or surgery. Injury of these vessels could cause catastrophic hemorrhage.

References

Ralls PW. Color Doppler sonography of the hepatic artery and portal venous system. *AJR* 1990;155:517–525.
Zwiebel WJ. Sonographic diagnosis of hepatic vascular disorders. *Semin Ultraound CT MR* 1995;16:34–48.

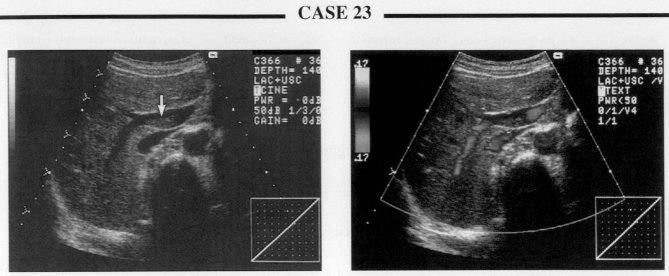

FIG. 52A. Grayscale.

FIG. 52B. Color Doppler.

History

A 39-year-old cirrhotic male with an elevated α-protein level. Sonography of the liver was performed to evaluate the possibility of hepatocellular carcinoma.

Findings

Figure 52A is a transverse grayscale sonogram showing a thrombus (arrow) of medium echogenicity in the pre-bifurcation right portal vein. Figure 52B is a color Doppler sonogram revealing that the clot is only partially echogenic; there is an anechoic portion. The clot is only partially occlusive, as there is flow seen in the anterior and posterior segmental branches distal to the partially occlusive thrombus.

Diagnosis

Right portal vein thrombosis.

Discussion

Portal vein thrombosis in portal hypertension is not rare: the prevalence in some series is as high as 15%. Nonneoplastic thrombus, as in this case, may be totally anechoic and invisible on grayscale images. The grayscale sonogram underestimated the extent of the clot in this patient. The diagnosis of portal venous thrombus was, nevertheless, evident from the grayscale image. No liver neoplasm was detected sonographically or on a subsequent CT scan.

References

Ralls PW. Color Doppler sonography of the hepatic artery and portal venous system. *AJR* 1990;155:517–525.
Zwiebel WJ. Sonographic diagnosis of hepatic vascular disorders. *Semin Ultrasound CT MR* 1995;16:34–48.

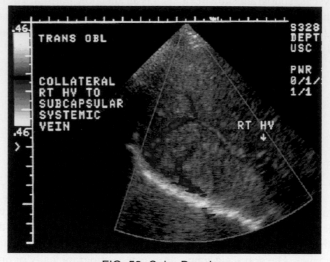

FIG. 53. Color Doppler.

History

A 9-year-old female with abnormal liver function test results who had normal contrast CT, MRI, and grayscale ultrasound results at an another hospital. She was referred to our hospital for an hepatic color Doppler sonogram.

Findings

Figure 53, an oblique transverse sonogram through the cephalic portion of the liver, shows flow in an hepatic vein toward the inferior vena cava (coded blue). This hepatic vein, however, does not empty normally into the inferior vena cava. Rather, an hepatic venous collateral (coded red) in which blood is flowing away from the liver is noted. This collateral feeds other hepatic venous collaterals (coded blue) that communicate with subcapsular hepatic veins. This blue-and-red V-shaped hepatic vein configuration is nearly diagnostic for hepatic venous collaterals associated with Budd–Chiari syndrome.

Diagnosis

Budd–Chiari syndrome.

Discussion

Budd–Chiari syndrome occurs when there is blockage of the normal egress of blood from the liver via the hepatic veins. Communication of peripheral hepatic veins to subcapsular systemic vein collaterals is one of the two major ways in which blood can exit the liver in patients with Budd–Chiari syndrome. The other is by portosystemic collaterals, usually via paraumbilical collaterals.

References

Jeffrey RB Jr, Ralls PW. The liver. In: *CT and sonography of the acute abdomen.* 2nd ed. Philadelphia: Lippincott–Raven, 1996:50–54.

Ralls PW, Johnson MB, Radin DR, et al. Budd–Chiari syndrome: detection with color Doppler sonography. *AJR* 1992;159:113–116.

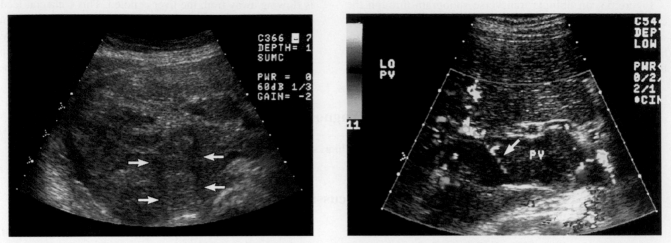

FIG. 54A. Grayscale.

FIG. 54B. Color Doppler.

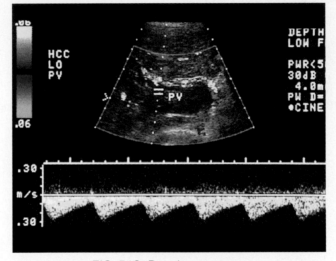

FIG. 54C. Doppler spectrum.

History

A 44-year-old alcoholic male with malaise, weight loss, and right upper-quadrant pain.

Findings

Figure 54A, a transverse grayscale scan of the right lobe of the liver, demonstrates marked parenchymal heterogeneity and a small amount of perihepatic ascites. Note the refractive shadow emanating centrally from the right lobe consistent with a space-occupying mass (arrows). Figures 54B and C are color Doppler sonograms of a portal vein thrombus that demonstrate arterial flow on color and spectral Doppler (arrow, Fig. 54C). Note that the direction of arterial flow is hepatofugal.

Diagnosis

Hepatocellular carcinoma with invasion of the portal vein.

Discussion

Parenchymal heterogeneity on grayscale imaging is a nonspecific finding and may be caused by cirrhosis, fatty infiltration, or tumor. The identification of a refractive shadow, however, strongly suggests the presence of an underlying hepatic mass, which proved to be due to hepatocellular carcinoma. Color Doppler imaging clearly facilitated detection of portal venous tumor invasion in this patient with a hepatoma. In selected patients with tumor neovascularity, arterial flow can be identified with color Doppler imaging of the thrombus. Characteristically, the arterial flow extends in a retrograde (hepatofugal) fashion down the portal vein toward the hepatic hilum. The finding of arterial flow is specific for tumor neovascularity and definitely precludes surgical resection for cure. The sensitivity of this finding is rather low, although the specificity for tumor invasion is high. In patients with suspected tumor invasion of the portal vein, but without color flow within the thrombus, fine-needle aspiration biopsy may be useful to confirm tumor thrombus. This finding is associated with a very poor prognosis.

References

Dodd GD III, Memel DS, Baron RL, Eichner L, Santguida LA. Portal vein thrombosis in patients with cirrhosis: does sonographic detection of intrathrombus flow allow differentiation of benign and malignant thrombus? *AJR* 1995;165:573–578.

Tanaka K, Numata K, Okazaki H, Nakamura S, Inoue S, Takamura Y. Diagnosis of portal vein thrombosis in patients with hepatocellular carcinoma: efficacy of color Doppler sonography compared with angiography. *AJR* 1993;160:1279–1283.

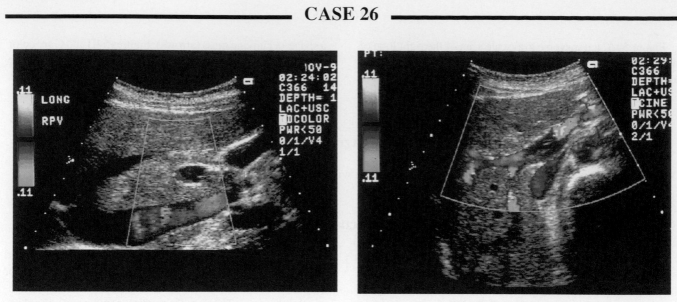

FIG. 55A. Color Doppler.

FIG. 55B. Color Doppler.

History

A 43-year-old alcoholic male with vague right upper-quadrant pain.

Findings

Figure 55A, a color Doppler sonogram through the right portal vein, reveals an area of no flow in the pre-bifurcation in the right portal vein. Note the flow in the anterior and posterior segmental branches distal to the apparently complete thrombus. Figure 55B, a longitudinal color Doppler sonogram through the portal vein, reveals a small, persistent flow channel representing a partial portal venous clot.

Diagnosis

Partial right portal vein clot.

Discussion

Portal vein thrombosis is a not uncommon occurrence in patients with portal hypertension. Color Doppler sonography is ideally suited to diagnose partial portal venous thrombus. This hypoechoic to anechoic thrombus was not detected on grayscale imaging. The cross-sectional view through the pre-bifurcation portal vein showed a small, persistent flow channel, explaining the presence of flow in the segmental branches of the right portal vein beyond the apparently occlusive thrombus. This information is available at a glance with color flow techniques. Grayscale with spectral Doppler would be much less likely to provide a clear picture of the true situation.

Reference

Ralls PW. Color Doppler sonography of the hepatic artery and portal venous system. *AJR* 1990;155:517–525.

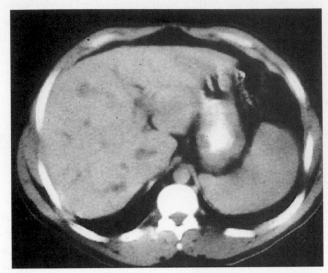

FIG. 56A. Noncontrast CT.

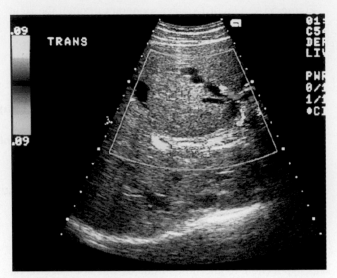

FIG. 56B. Color Doppler.

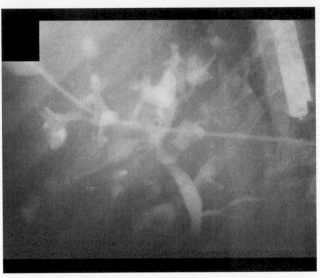

FIG. 56C. Endoscopic retrograde cholangiopancreatography.

History

A 39-year-old male with intermittent jaundice.

Findings

Figure 56A is a noncontrast CT scan showing low-attenuation areas of uncertain etiology in the liver. Figure 56B, a transverse color Doppler sonogram in the region of the left and right portal vein, reveals multiple dilated cystic areas that communicate with the intrahepatic bile ducts. Figure 56C is an endoscopic retrograde cholangiopancreatography demonstrating the same cystic dilatation of the intrahepatic bile ducts.

Diagnosis

Caroli's disease.

Discussion

Caroli's disease, a cystic dilatation of the intrahepatic bile ducts, was originally described as being characterized by saccular dilatation of these ducts, with a predisposition to biliary stone disease, cholangitis, and liver abscess, and an association with renal cystic disease. A review by Barros et al. revealed that there is a spectrum of associated findings. Some cases have hepatic fibrosis and portal hypertension (similar to congenital hepatic fibrosis), whereas others are associated with a choledochal cyst (Todani type 4A). To call an isolated intrahepatic cyst a "type 5" choledochal cyst is probably inappropriate. Thus, Caroli's disease is probably several separate entities. Those patients with congenital hepatic fibrosis (of which infantile polycystic kidney disease is part of the spectrum) have a high prevalence of renal cysts and markedly dilated renal tubules (tubular ectasia) and may have complications of portal hypertension (such as gastrointestinal bleeds). The prevalence of cholangiocarcinoma is ~7%, or 100 times higher than in the general population.

References

Barros JL, Polo JR, Sanabia J, et al. Congenital cystic dilatation of the intrahepatic bile ducts (Caroli's disease). *Surgery* 1979;85:589–592.

Shulte SJ. Embryology, normal variation, and congenital anomalies of the gallbladder and biliary tract. In: Freeny PC, Stevenson GW, eds. *Margolis & Burhenne's alimentary tract radiology*. St. Louis: CV Mosby, 1994.

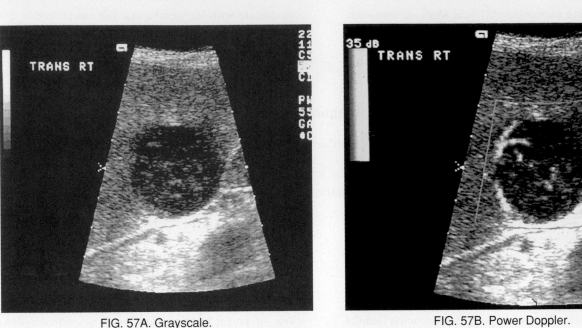

FIG. 57A. Grayscale.

FIG. 57B. Power Doppler.

History

A 38-year-old female with HIV infection who had abnormal liver function test results and vague upper abdominal pain. An hepatic ultrasound was ordered.

Findings

Figure 57A, a transverse grayscale sonogram in the upper abdomen near the inferior vena cava, reveals a mainly hypoechoic, ~3 cm mass with some internal heterogeneity. Figure 57B, a power Doppler image of this lesion, shows increased peripheral flow with some internal flow. Flow from the contiguous inferior vena cava, which is essentially invisible on the grayscale image, is seen here, adjacent to the lesion.

Diagnosis

AIDS lymphoma of the liver.

Discussion

Moderate- to high-grade B-cell lymphoma in an HIV-positive patient is an AIDS-defining condition, whereas other non-Hodgkin's lymphoma and Hodgkin's lymphoma are not AIDS-defining conditions. AIDS-related B-cell lymphomas are very aggressive and should be considered disseminated at presentation, even when only local disease is evident. Primary gastric and primary CNS lymphoma are common in AIDS patients. Parenchymal disease in most lymphomas is infiltrative and thus difficult to image. Focal disease is common in AIDS-related lymphoma, distinct from other lymphomas. Focal lesions involving the liver, spleen, adrenals, and kidneys are common. AIDS-related lymphomas often can be treated successfully with relatively mild chemotherapeutic regimens. Although early and extensive recurrence is common, many patients do not die of lymphoma, but rather of some other AIDS-related condition.

Reference

Radin DR, Esplin JA, Levine AM, et al. AIDS-related non-Hodgkin's lymphoma: abdominal CT findings in 112 patients. *AJR* 1993;160:1133-1139.

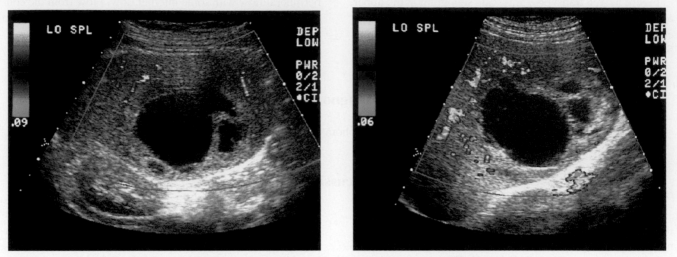

FIG. 58A. Color Doppler.

FIG. 58B. Color Doppler.

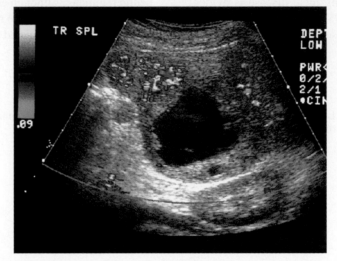

FIG. 58C. Color Doppler.

History

A 64-year-old female with known nasopharyngeal carcinoma who had vague left upper-quadrant pain.

Findings

Figures 58A–C are longitudinal and transverse scans of the spleen that demonstrate a complex cystic mass containing vascularized solid components.

Diagnosis

Cystic metastasis to the spleen from nasopharyngeal carcinoma.

Discussion

Cystic lesions of the spleen include congenital cysts, acquired cystic lesions (i.e., cystic pancreatic pseudocysts and old hematomas from trauma), and primary or metastatic neoplasms. The most common neoplasms to involve the spleen include lymphoma, melanoma, and carcinoma, particularly ovarian carcinoma. Other causes of cystic splenic lesions include parasitic cysts and abscesses, although the clinical presentation is much different than with neoplasm. Fine-needle aspiration biopsy performed along the solid rim of the complex cystic mass under ultrasound control confirmed the nasopharyngeal carcinoma. The patient was treated with chemotherapy, but died of widespread metastases 5 months later. The key feature suggesting a splenic neoplasm was the identification of vascularized solid components in the predominantly cystic mass. Although lymphoma is the most common neoplasm to involve the spleen, it is rarely cystic.

Reference

Ha HK, Kim HH, Kim BK, Han JK, Choi BI. Primary angiosarcoma of the spleen: CT and MR imaging. *Acta Radiol* 1994;35:455–458.

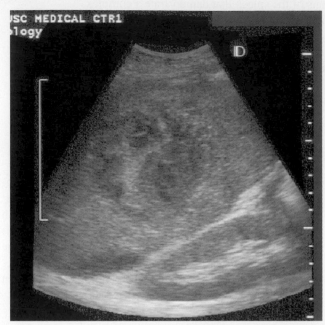

FIG. 59A. Grayscale.

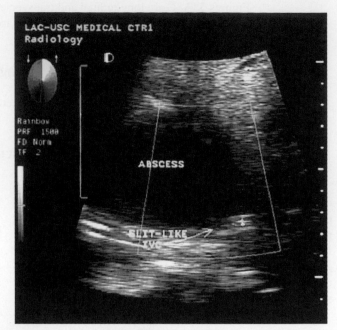

FIG. 59B. Color Doppler.

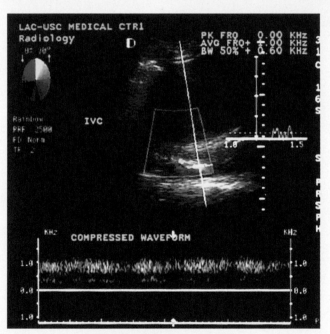

FIG. 59C. Doppler spectrum.

History

A 36-year-old male with pain, fever, and a right upper-quadrant mass.

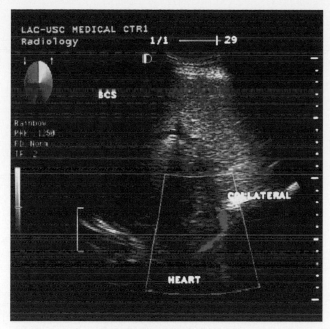

FIG. 59D. Color Doppler.

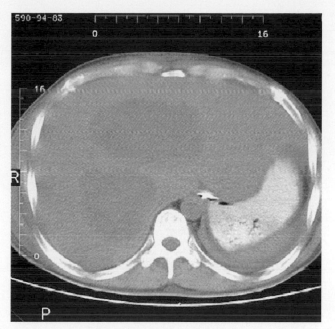

FIG. 59E. Noncontrast CT.

Findings

Figure 59A, a longitudinal sonogram through the right lobe of the liver, shows a heterogeneous mass in the right lobe that, because of elevated amebic titers, was determined to be an amebic liver abscess. Figure 59B is a transverse color Doppler sonogram that shows narrowing of the inferior vena cava by the mass producing a flat, so-called compressed waveform in the spectral Doppler image below the level of the inferior vena caval obstruction (Fig. 59C). Figure 59D, a color Doppler sonogram in the cephalic liver, reveals a hepatic venous to pericardio-cardiophrenic vein collateral. This peripheral hepatic venous to systemic venous collateral makes the diagnosis of Budd–Chiari syndrome likely. Figure 59E is a noncontrast CT confirming the presence of multiple amebic liver abscesses. Because these lesions were associated with Budd–Chiari syndrome in this patient, percutaneous drainage was performed.

Diagnosis

Budd–Chiari syndrome secondary to amebic liver abscess.

Discussion

Hepatic veins may occasionally be compressed in patients with hepatic amebic abscess. Although this is uncommon in the Western hemisphere, it is reportedly common in India.

References

Jeffrey RB Jr, Ralls PW. The liver. In: *CT and sonography of the acute abdomen.* 2nd ed. Philadelphia: Lippincott–Raven, 1996:50–54.

Ralls PW, Johnson MB, Radin DR, et al. Budd–Chiari syndrome: detection with color Doppler sonography. *AJR* 1992;159:113–116.

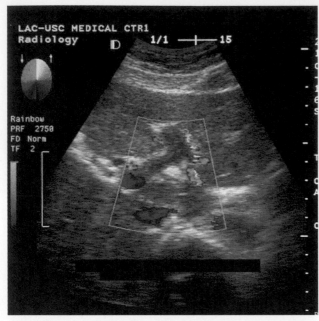

FIG. 60A. Color Doppler.

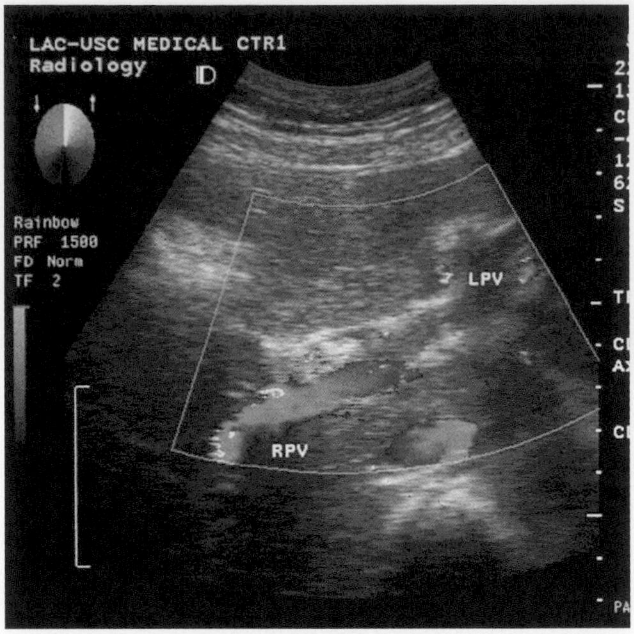

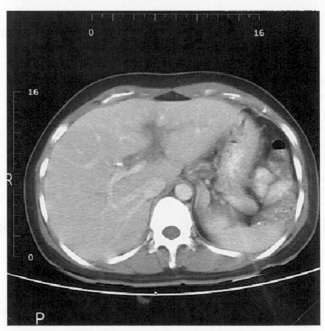

FIG. 60B. Color Doppler.

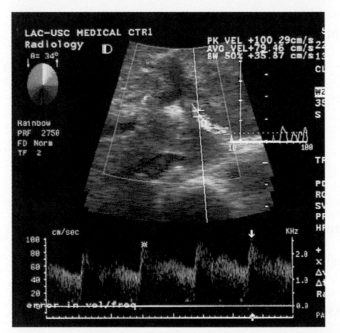

FIG. 60C. Doppler spectrum.

FIG. 60D. Contrast-enhanced CT.

History

A 31-year-old female with right lower-quadrant pain who underwent open appendectomy. Several days later, her fever recurred, and she developed an elevated white blood cell count, with right upper-quadrant pain. Abdominal sonography and hepatic sonography were requested.

Findings

Figures 60A and B are transverse color Doppler sonograms revealing complete thrombosis of the proximal and distal left portal vein. Note the replaced left hepatic artery in the fissure for ligamentum venosum. Figure 60C is a color Doppler-guided spectral Doppler sonogram showing arterial flow within the replaced left hepatic artery in the fissure for ligamentum venosum. The left hepatic artery often arises (~25%) from the left gastric artery and enters the liver via the fissure for the ligamentum venosum, as in this case. Figure 60D is a contrast-enhanced CT confirming the sonographic findings of portal vein occlusion (pylephlebitis septic portal venous thrombosis). The CT was performed because sonography failed to demonstrate an hepatic abscess. Hepatic abscess is a common complication of pylephlebitis. CT also failed to identify a focal hepatic abscess.

Diagnosis

Pylephlebitis from appendicitis.

Discussion

Ascending infection via the portal system is pylephlebitis. Portal venous sepsis usually arises from a gastrointestinal focus, often appendicitis, as in this case. The term *pylephlebitis* is generally used when there is associated portal venous clot. Thrombus can be confidently diagnosed with color Doppler when no flow is seen within the vessel and flow is seen in other vessels at the same depth and in the same field of view. The diagnosis is facilitated when echogenic material is found within the vessel, as in this case. Anechoic thrombus, frequently occurring in nonmalignant thrombosis, may also be diagnosed reliably by using these criteria. Care must be taken to ensure that all technical parameters are considered appropriately. Septic portal thrombosis and pylephlebitis may occur subsequently to gastrointestinal infection, especially diverticulitis and appendicitis. Occasionally, other conditions may cause pylephlebitis. Liver abscess is a common complication of pylephlebitis. Liver abscesses, formerly thought almost universally fatal, are really no more difficult to treat than pyogenic liver abscesses of other etiologies.

References

Jeffrey RB Jr, Ralls PW. The liver. In: *CT and sonography of the acute abdomen*. 2nd ed. Philadelphia: Lippincott–Raven, 1996:62–65.

Lim GM, Jeffrey RB Jr, Ralls PW, et al. Septic thrombosis of the portal vein: CT and clinical observations. *J Comput Assist Tomogr* 1989;13:656–658.

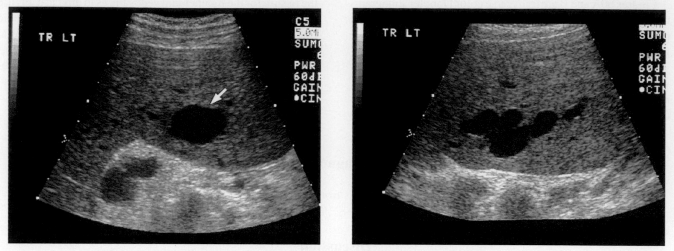

FIG. 61A. Grayscale.

FIG. 61B. Grayscale.

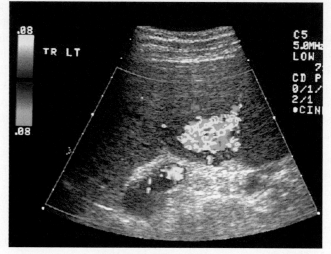

FIG. 61C. Color Doppler.

History

A 33-year-old male with Crohn's disease who, 8 months after pelvic abscess drainage, developed splenomegaly.

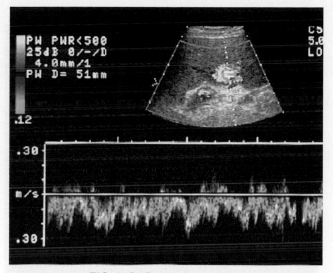

FIG. 61D. Doppler spectrum.

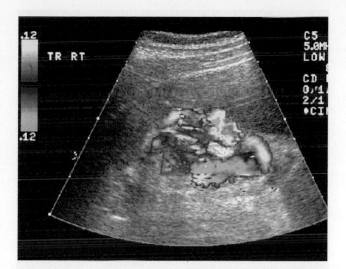

FIG. 61E. Color Doppler.

Findings

Figure 61A, a transverse scan of the left lobe of the liver, demonstrates a cystic mass (arrow). Note in Fig. 61B, which is also a grayscale image, that several branching hypoechoic structures are emanating from the cystic mass. Figure 61C is a color Doppler sonogram demonstrating the vascular nature of the mass. A spectral Doppler tracing (Fig. 61D) demonstrates venous flow within this lesion consistent with a venous aneurysm. Figure 61E, a transverse scan of the porta hepatis, demonstrates numerous color-coded venous collaterals caused by cavernous transformation of the portal vein.

Diagnosis

Cavernous transformation of the portal vein with an intrahepatic portal venous aneurysm.

Discussion

Cavernous transformation in this patient with Crohn's disease was likely caused by septic thrombosis of the portal vein from a prior pelvic abscess. Extensive venous collaterals developed in the porta hepatis. Intrahepatic venous collaterals resulted in an intrahepatic portal venous aneurysm. Venous aneurysms are rare and most often noted in the internal jugular, popliteal, and portal veins. Some cases are related to a portal vein to hepatic vein fistula. Portal venous aneurysms are of no clinical consequence and do not result in any significant morbidity. Color Doppler can aid in avoiding misdiagnosis, such as confusing a portal venous aneurysm with a complex fluid collection such as an abscess.

References

Calligaro KD, Ahmad S, Dandor R, et al. Venous aneurysms: surgical indications and review of the literature. *Surgery* 1995;117:1 6.

Tanaka K, Numata K, Okazaki H, Nakamura S, Inoue S, Takamura Y. Diagnosis of portal vein thrombosis in patients with hepatocellular carcinoma: efficacy of color Doppler sonography compared with angiography. *AJR* 1993;160:1279–1283.

Tarazov PG. Spontaneous aneurysmal intrahepatic portosystemic venous shunt. *Cardiovasc Intervent Radiol* 1994; 17:44–45.

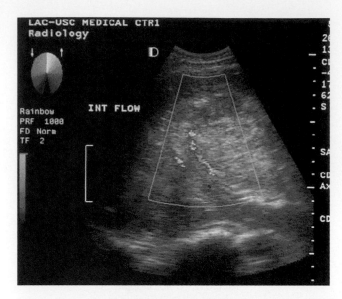

FIG. 62A. Color Doppler.

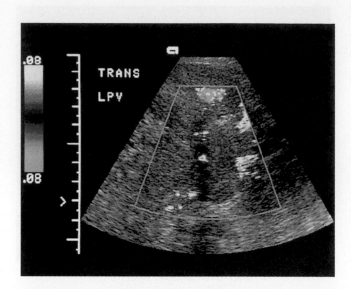

FIG. 62B. Color Doppler.

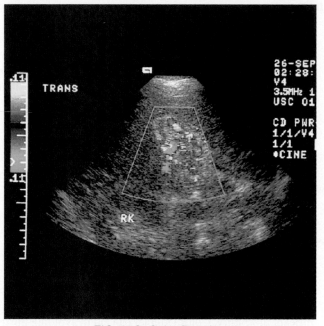

FIG. 62C. Color Doppler.

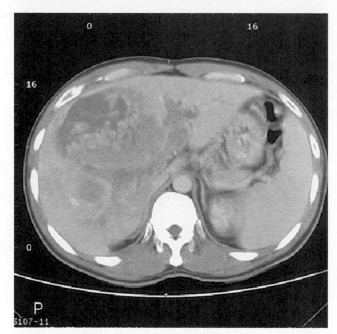

FIG. 62D. Contrast-enhanced CT.

History

A 36-year-old male with chronic hepatitis B who was in pain and had an upper abdominal mass. Ultrasound was used to evaluate the mass.

Findings

Figure 62A, a sagittal oblique image through the liver, shows a large hepatocellular cancer with internal color flow. A thrombosed portal vein is noted. Complete thrombosis of the entire portal venous system was documented sonographically. Figure 62B, an enlarged image of the thrombosed left portal vein, reveals internal flow within the tumor thrombus. Flow within the thrombus is strongly suggestive of venous invasion by neoplasm. Figure 62C is color Doppler that shows gallbladder wall varices, which generally occur when there is portal vein thrombosis. With portal vein thrombosis, hepatopedal collaterals form. When the veins in the gallbladder wall are recruited, gallbladder wall varices result. Figure 62D is a contrast-enhanced CT showing a large, multilobulated mass involving both the left and right lobes with variable patterns of enhancement. The left and right portal veins are involved by tumor thrombus.

Diagnosis

Hepatocellular cancer with portal vein occlusion and gallbladder wall varices.

Discussion

Hepatocellular cancer is a well-known complication of chronic hepatitis-B infection that may occur even in a patient this young. The sonogram confirmed the clinical suspicion of hepatocellular cancer and documented flow within the tumor mass. Color Doppler flow is present in 75% to 80% of all hepatocellular cancers. Portal venous thrombosis from tumor invasion is also common.

References

Nino-Murcia M, Ralls PW, Jeffrey RB Jr, et al. Color flow Doppler characterization of focal hepatic lesions. *AJR* 1992;159:1195–1197.

Stephens DH, Johnson CD. Primary malignant neoplasms of the liver. In: Freeny PC, Stevenson GW, eds. *Margolis & Burhenne's alimentary tract radiology*. St. Louis: CV Mosby, 1994.

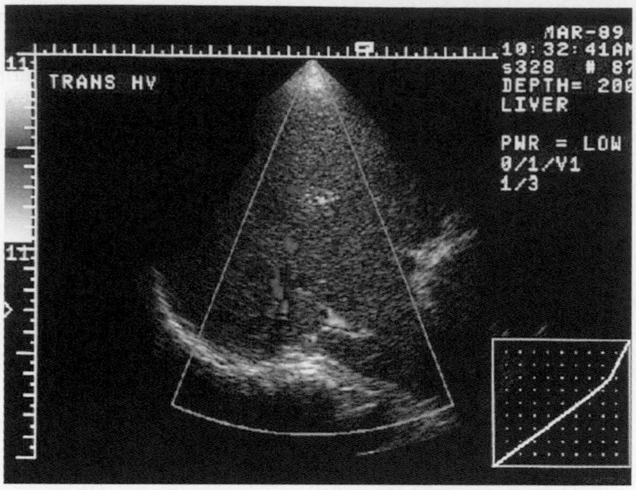

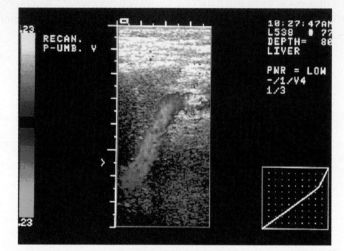

FIG. 63A. Color Doppler.

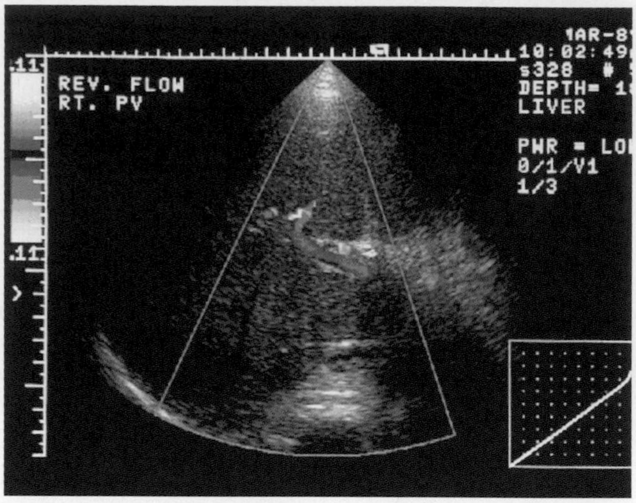

FIG. 63B. Color Doppler.

FIG. 63C. Color Doppler.

History

A 53-year-old male with vague right upper-quadrant pain.

Findings

Figure 63A is a transverse color Doppler sonogram showing no normal hepatic veins entering the inferior vena cava. A tortuous narrowed hepatic venous collateral enters the inferior vena cava from its dorsal aspect. Figure 63B is a transverse color Doppler sonogram showing flow reversal (flow away from the liver periphery) in the right portal vein. Figure 63C is a longitudinal color Doppler sonogram revealing a recanalized paraumbilical vein.

Diagnosis

Budd–Chiari syndrome, decompressed via a recanalized paraumbilical vein.

Discussion

Budd–Chiari syndrome occurs when there is blockage of the normal egress of blood from the liver via the hepatic veins. Portosystemic collaterals, usually via paraumbilical collaterals, is the most common pathway in patients with Budd–Chiari syndrome. Communication of peripheral hepatic veins to subcapsular systemic venous collaterals is the other common type of collateralization.

References

Jeffrey RB Jr, Ralls PW. The liver. In: *CT and sonography of the acute abdomen.* 2nd ed. Philadelphia: Lippincott–Raven, 1996:50–54.

Ralls PW, Johnson MB, Radin DR, et al. Budd–Chiari syndrome: detection with color Doppler sonography. *AJR* 1992;159:113–116.

Section 3

The Gallbladder and Bile Ducts

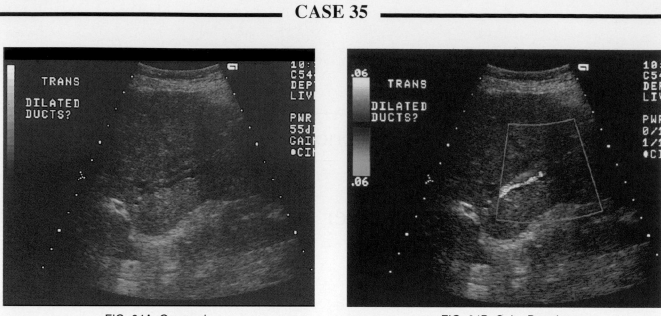

FIG. 64A. Grayscale.　　　　　　　　FIG. 64B. Color Doppler.

History

A 42-year-old male with jaundice and alcoholic liver disease who was referred for sonography.

Findings

Figure 64A is a transverse sonogram of the lateral segment of the left lobe. There are parallel anechoic tubular structures seen in the lateral segment, suggesting the possibility of dilated bile ducts. Figure 64B, a color Doppler sonogram in the same region, reveals flow in both of the anechoic channels. These anechoic structures are vascular and not a dilated intrahepatic duct with its accompanying vessel.

Diagnosis

False-positive double-channel sign simulating biliary dilatation.

Discussion

This patient has chronic active hepatitis. The increased arterial flow that occurs in this condition often results in enlarged, high-flow arteries. Portal hypertension may result in smaller portal veins, as in this case. There is flow reversal in the portal vein (the blue-coded vessel). The portal vein and accompanying enlarged artery (the dorsal vessel with aliased flow) may result in a grayscale appearance that simulates intrahepatic biliary ductal dilatation. Color Doppler reveals the true situation at a glance, preventing a false-positive diagnosis for bile duct dilatation.

Reference

Ralls PW. Color Doppler sonography of the hepatic artery and portal venous system. *AJR* 1990:155:517–525.

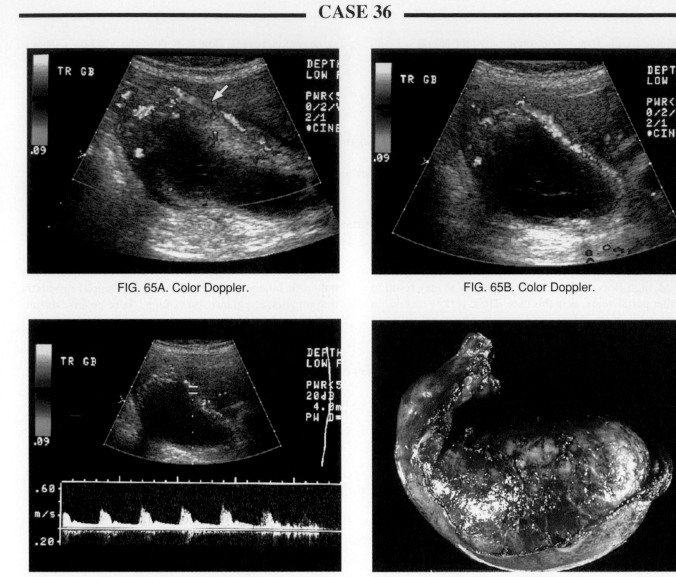

FIG. 65A. Color Doppler.

FIG. 65B. Color Doppler.

FIG. 65C. Doppler spectrum.

FIG. 65D. Pathology specimen.

History

A 72-year-old female with fever and mid-epigastric pain.

Findings

Figures 65A and B are color Doppler sonograms of the gallbladder that demonstrate marked hypertrophy of the cystic artery (arrow, Fig. 65A) with prominent flow in the gallbladder fundus. Note the gallstones, intraluminal membranes, mural thickening, and subtle pericholecystic fluid in Fig. 65A. Figure 65C is a spectral Doppler tracing that confirms arterial flow within the cystic artery. Figure 65D shows a pathologic specimen demonstrating gangrenous cholecystitis.

Diagnosis

Color Doppler sonography of gangrenous cholecystitis.

Discussion

Of interest in this patient was the fact that there was no evidence of a sonographic Murphy's sign, because there was no focal tenderness directly over the gallbladder. This finding may be absent in up to one-third of patients with gangrenous cholecystitis, because transmural infarction of the gallbladder wall results in necrosis of the afferent nerve fibers innervating the gallbladder. In normal patients, the cystic artery can be identified with color Doppler sonography using low-volume flow sensitivity in ~50% of patients. Generally, the anterior division of the cystic artery is visualized near the neck of the gallbladder. It is exceedingly rare for the cystic artery to be visualized in the distal fundal quartile of the gallbladder, and thus flow in this area on color Doppler strongly suggests hyperemia from inflammation. Most patients with acute cholecystitis will not demonstrate an abnormal flow pattern of the cystic artery in the gallbladder wall. This is more common in patients with more advanced inflammation such as gangrenous cholecystitis.

References

Jeffrey RB Jr, Nino-Murcia M, Ralls PW, Jain KA, Davidson HC. Color Doppler sonography of the cystic artery: comparison of normal controls and patients with acute cholecystitis. *J Ultrasound Med* 1995;14:33–36.

Lee FT Jr, DeLone DR, Bean DW, et al. Acute cholecystitis in an animal model: findings on color Doppler sonography. *AJR* 1995;165:85–90.

McDonnell CH III, Jeffrey RB Jr, Vierra MA. Inflamed pericholecystic fat: color Doppler flow imaging and clinical features. *Radiology* 1994;193:547–550.

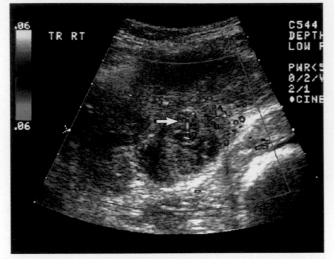

FIG. 66A. Color Doppler.

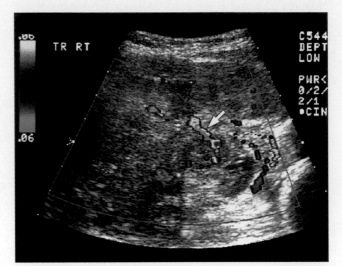

FIG. 66B. Color Doppler.

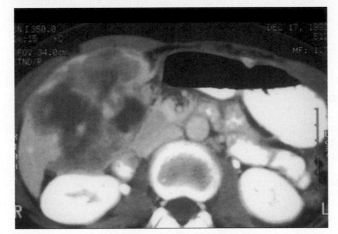

FIG. 66C. Contrast-enhanced CT.

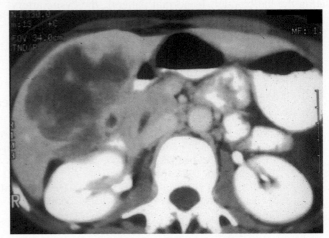

FIG. 66D. Contrast-enhanced CT.

History

A 38-year-old female with intermittent right upper-quadrant pain. Rule out gallstones.

Findings

Figures 66A and B are transverse color Doppler sonograms of the gallbladder and liver. Note that the echogenic tissue within the gallbladder has vascular flow identified with color Doppler sonography (arrows). Figures 66C and D are contrast-enhanced CT scans that demonstrate a large low-attenuation mass originating from the gallbladder and directly invading the adjacent liver.

Diagnosis

Gallbladder carcinoma with direct hepatic invasion.

Discussion

Internal echoes within the lumen of the gallbladder are most often caused by sludge, hemorrhage, or pus, all of which are avascular on color Doppler sonography. The echogenic tissue in this patient demonstrated clear-cut evidence of flow, indicating that it represented a solid mass. Although somewhat subtle on the grayscale images, there was marked heterogeneity of the adjacent hepatic parenchyma. The extent of the tumor was much more clearly demonstrated on the contrast-enhanced CT because the low-density areas of direct invasion were clearly evident. This patient had a rapid downhill course and died within 3 months of the diagnosis. Gallbladder carcinoma is quite unusual in young patients and in patients without obvious gallstones. A fine-needle aspiration biopsy of the liver lesions revealed adenocarcinoma consistent with a primary gallbladder tumor. Direct hepatic invasion generally precludes surgical resection for cure and has a dismal prognosis.

References

Franquet T, Montes M, Ruiz de Azua Y, Jimenez FJ, Cozcolluela R. Primary gallbladder carcinoma: imaging findings in 50 patients with pathologic correlation. *Gastrointest Radiol* 1991;16:143–148.

Suminski N, Johnson MB, Ralls PW. Color Doppler sonography in gallbladder carcinoma. *J Clin Ultrasound* 1991; 19:183–186.

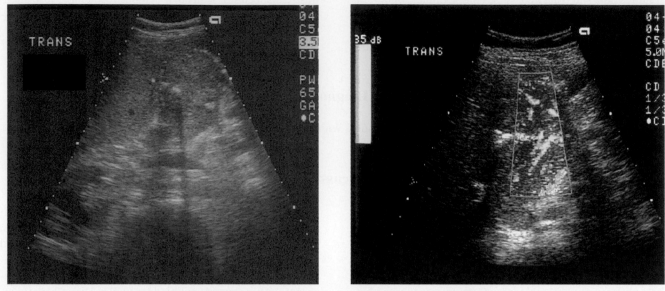

FIG. 67A. Grayscale.   FIG. 67B. Power Doppler.

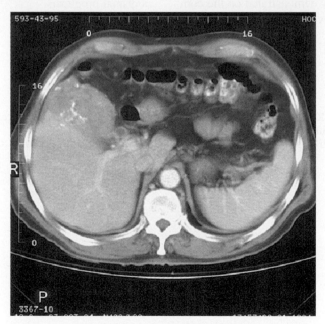

FIG. 67C. Contrast-enhanced CT.

History

A 61-year-old male with right upper-quadrant pain and fatty-food intolerance who was referred for right upper-quadrant sonography to rule out cholelithiasis.

Findings

Figure 67A, a transverse sonogram of the gallbladder, shows multiple calcifications in the wall of the gallbladder and within the gallbladder itself. Within the gallbladder is an inhomogeneous soft tissue mass. Figure 67B is a power Doppler sonogram showing extensive flow within the gall-bladder mass and calcifications present within the mass. Gallbladder carcinoma was diagnosed. Figure 67C, a contrast-enhanced CT scan showing the mural calcifications in the mass within the gallbladder, confirms the diagnosis.

Diagnosis

Porcelain gallbladder with gallbladder carcinoma.

Discussion

The calcification in the gallbladder wall, the mass in the gallbladder, and the presence of flow within the mass virtually clinched the diagnosis of gallbladder carcinoma. Flow within a gallbladder mass is nearly diagnostic for gallbladder carcinoma, although not all gallbladder carcinomas have internal flow that can be imaged with color or power Doppler. There is a high prevalence of gallbladder carcinoma in patients with porcelain gallbladder (mural gallbladder calcification).

Reference

Suminski N, Johnson MB, Ralls PW. Color Doppler sonography in gallbladder carcinoma. *J Clin Ultrasound* 1991;19:183–186.

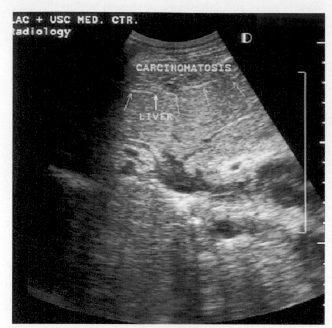

FIG. 68A. Grayscale.

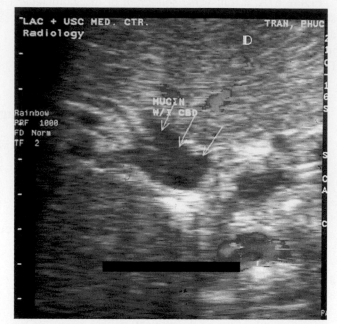

FIG. 68B. Color Doppler.

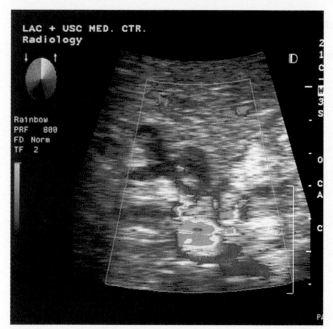

FIG. 68C. Color Doppler.

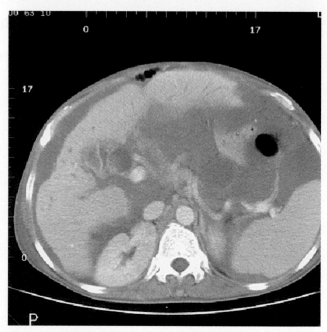

FIG. 68D. Contrast-enhanced CT.

History

A 63-year-old male with weight loss, jaundice, and abdominal distention.

Findings

Figure 68A, a sagittal sonogram near the region of the common duct, shows abnormal tissue superficial to the liver. This represents peritoneal carcinomatosis. Note the amorphous material within the bile ducts. Figure 68B, a longitudinal sonogram of the dilated bile duct system, shows a castlike, intermediate-level echogenic area within the bile duct. This is mucin produced by the mucinous cholangiocarcinoma (adenocarcinoma of the bile duct). Figure 68C, a longitudinal image slightly off axis from Fig. 68B, reveals flow within a nodular mass within the bile duct. Figure 68D is a contrast-enhanced CT scan showing carcinomatosis and heterogeneous material within the bile duct.

Diagnosis

Mucinous cholangiocarcinoma with carcinomatosis.

Discussion

This patient had advanced mucinous carcinomatosis, so-called pseudomyxoma peritonei. The findings of pseudomyxoma peritonei were shown best by the CT, but were also demonstrated by the sonogram. Although the findings within the bile duct were not specific for mucinous cholangiocarcinoma, a very rare lesion, the bile duct nodule with internal color flow suggested intraductal neoplasm. The amorphous, medium-level echogenicity material, representing intraductal mucin, suggested the correct diagnosis.

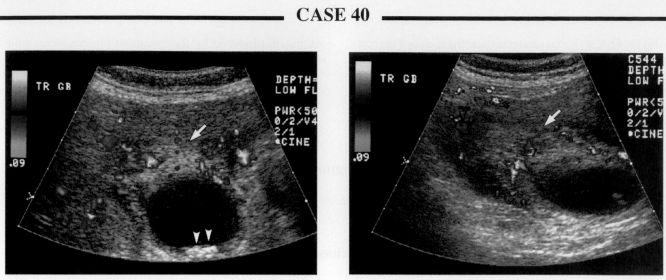

FIG. 69A. Color Doppler.   FIG. 69B. Color Doppler.

History

A 69-year-old female who had fever and right upper-quadrant tenderness for 1 week.

Findings

Figures 69A and B, transverse color Doppler sonograms of the gallbladder, demonstrate prominent echogenic tissue (arrows) that contains intrinsic vascularity. Small gallstones are seen in Fig. 69A (arrowheads).

Diagnosis

Acute cholecystitis with inflamed pericholecystic fat.

Discussion

Acute cholecystitis may cause edema and inflammation of the surrounding fat in the hepatoduodenal ligament and omentum. This is particularly true in cases of gangrenous cholecystitis, because there is transmural inflammation and a large surface area for contact with fat within ligaments and the omentum. In patients with gangrenous cholecystitis, the omentum acts to "seal off" perforations and prevent generalized peritonitis. As with inflamed fat elsewhere in the body, there is often increased echogenicity and increased flow on color Doppler imaging. This is a helpful finding that suggests gangrenous cholecystitis, as the patient did not have a sonographic Murphy sign.

References

Jeffrey RB Jr, Nino-Murcia M, Ralls PW, Jain KA, Davidson HC. Color Doppler sonography of the cystic artery: comparison of normal controls and patients with acute cholecystitis. *J Ultrasound Med* 1995;14:33–36.

McDonnell CH III, Jeffrey RB Jr, Vierra MA. Inflamed pericholecystic fat: color Doppler flow imaging and clinical features. *Radiology* 1994;193:547–550.

Paulson EK, Kliewer MA, Hertzberg BS. Diagnosis of acute cholecystitis with color Doppler sonography: significance of arterial flow in thickened gallbladder wall. *AJR* 1994;162:1105–1108.

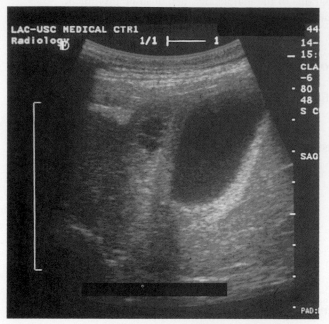

FIG. 70A. Grayscale.

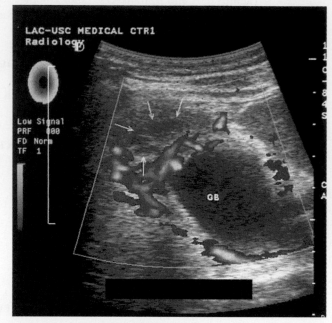

FIG. 70B. Power Doppler.

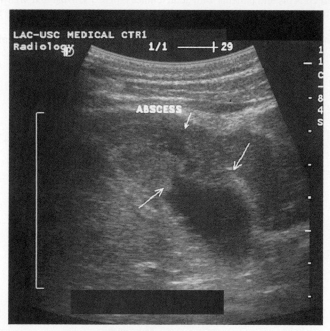

FIG. 70C. Grayscale.

History

A 38-year-old male with leukocytosis, fever, and right upper-quadrant pain. Sonography of the right upper quadrant was requested.

Findings

Figure 70A, a longitudinal oblique view of the gallbladder, reveals a multiseptated pericholecystic abscess contiguous to the gallbladder, which has a thickened wall. Figure 70B is a power Doppler image revealing mural hyperemia, as well as increased flow around the abscess. Figure 70C is a grayscale image showing interruption of the submucosa of the gallbladder wall, indicative of rupture in the region of the fundus.

Diagnosis

Acute cholecystitis with gallbladder rupture and pericholecystic abscess.

Discussion

Pericholecystic abscess is a common complication of severe acute cholecystitis. Severe hyperemia, as in this case, is a frequent finding in severe acute cholecystitis. In the correct clinical setting, fundal hyperemia, as in this case, and visualization of the cystic artery for >50% of the length of the gallbladder wall serve to suggest or confirm the diagnosis of acute cholecystitis. Gallbladder wall perforation is a necessary prerequisite to most pericholecystic abscesses. Interruption of the echogenic submucosa, demonstrated in this case, and hyperemia around pericholecystic abscesses are not always detected sonographically. When present, it supports the diagnosis of pericholecystic abscess. All sonographic findings were confirmed surgically.

References

Jeffrey RB Jr, Ralls PW. The gallbladder and bile ducts. In: *Sonography of the abdomen.* New York; Raven 1995:191.

Jeffrey RB Jr, Ralls PW. The gallbladder and bile ducts. In: *CT and sonography of the acute abdomen.* 2nd ed. Philadelphia: Lippincott–Raven, 1996:86–98.

SECTION 1

The Pancreas

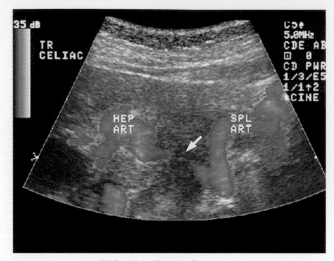

FIG. 71A. Power Doppler.

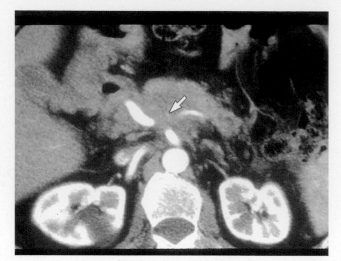

FIG. 71B. Contrast-enhanced CT.

History

A 71-year-old female with a 1-month history of mid-epigastric pain and normal endoscopic findings. Rule out biliary tract disease.

Findings

Figure 71A is a power Doppler sonogram of the celiac axis. Note the marked narrowing of the common hepatic artery (arrow). Figure 71B, a contrast-enhanced CT scan done 5 weeks later, demonstrates a large pancreatic mass that encases the celiac axis (arrow), causing compression and narrowing of both the hepatic and the splenic arteries.

Diagnosis

Pancreatic carcinoma encasing the hepatic artery.

Discussion

Unlike conventional color Doppler, power Doppler is much less angle dependent. With conventional color Doppler, no color signal is obtained at angles 90° to the ultrasound beam; therefore, it may be impossible to visualize flow within vessels perpendicular to the plane of the ultrasound beam. Power Doppler imaging is thus an excellent way to visualize horizontal branches of the celiac axis. In this case, the actual echogenicity of the tumor was difficult to differentiate from the that of liver and other surrounding tissues. However, the vascular encasement of the hepatic artery was obvious.

Arterial encasement from pancreatic carcinoma is uniformly associated with a poor outcome and precludes surgical resection for cure. A fine-needle biopsy performed under CT guidance revealed adenocarcinoma. The patient received radiation and chemotherapy, but died ~6 months after the CT scan. Both color and power Doppler are excellent techniques for diagnosing vascular extension of a pancreatic carcinoma. Venous occlusion and arterial encasement are often readily apparent with color or power Doppler imaging.

References

Bude RO, Rubin JM, Adler RS. Power versus conventional color Doppler sonography: comparison in the depiction of normal intrarenal vasculature. *Radiology* 1994;192:777–780.

Rubin JM, Bude RO, Carson PL, Bree RL, Adler RS. Power Doppler US: a potentially useful alternative to mean frequency based color Doppler US. *Radiology* 1994;190:853–856.

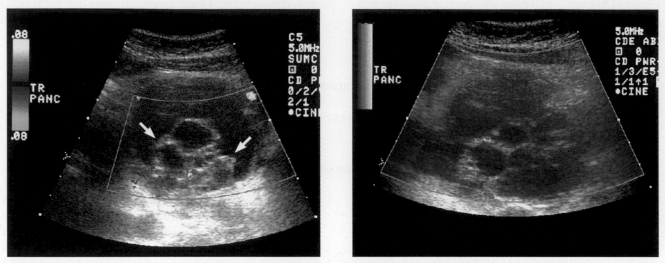

FIG. 72A. Color Doppler.　　　　　　　　　　FIG. 72B. Power Doppler.

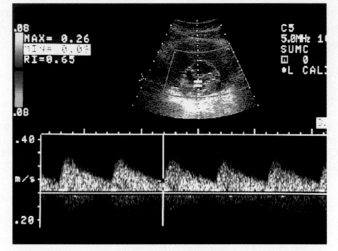

FIG. 72C. Doppler spectrum.

History

A 42-year-old female with vague mid-epigastric pain. Rule out gallbladder disease.

Findings

Figures 72A and B are color and power Doppler sonograms of the tail of the pancreas that demonstrate a complex cystic mass (arrows) with septations and internal vascular flow. The spec- tral Doppler tracing (Fig. 72C) reveals arterial flow with a high diastolic component within the septae.

Diagnosis

Mucinous cystadenocarcinoma of the pancreas.

Discussion

The differential diagnosis of complex cystic masses orig- inating from the pancreas includes hemorrhagic or infected pseudocysts and necrotic primary or metastatic cystic neo- plasms of the pancreas. The vascularized septations within the mass strongly suggested a diagnosis of neoplasm, most likely a primary mucinous cystadenocarcinoma. Unlike mi- crocystic adenomas, which are almost universally benign, these "macrocystic" lesions have high malignant potential and usually present with symptoms of mass effect because of the largeness of the lesion. The locules are considerably larger than with the microcystic variety, which is perhaps the most useful differentiating feature.

References

Hammel P, Levy P, Voitot H, et al. Preoperative cyst fluid analysis is useful for the differential diagnosis of cys- tic lesions of the pancreas. *Gastroenterology* 1995;108:1230–1235.

Healy JC, Davies SE, Reznek RH. CT of microcystic (serous) pancreatic adenoma. *J Comput Assist Tomogr* 1994, 18:146–148.

Padovani B, Mouvout P, Chanalet S, et al. Microcystic adenoma of the pancreas: report on four cases and review of the literature. *Gastrointest Radiol* 1991;16:62–66.

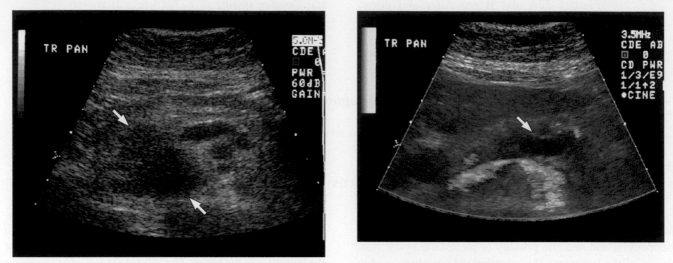

FIG. 73A. Grayscale.

FIG. 73B. Power Doppler.

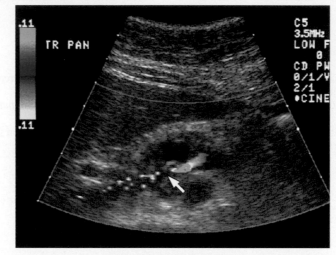

FIG. 73C. Color Doppler.

History

A 74-year-old male who had mid-epigastric pain for 2 months and a 15-pound weight loss.

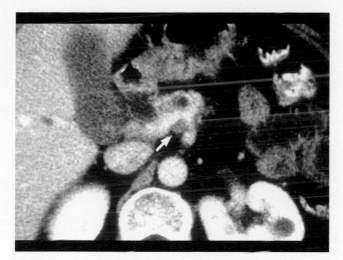

FIG. 73D. Contrast-enhanced CT.

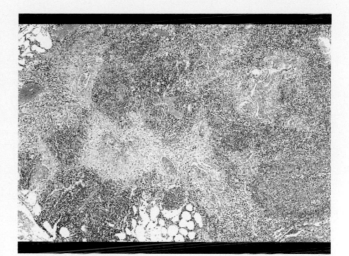

FIG. 73E. Pathology slide.

Findings

Figure 73A, a transverse grayscale image of the pancreas, demonstrates a large hypoechoic mass (arrows) involving the head and neck of the pancreas. Note the dilatation of the main pancreatic duct (arrow) adjacent to the mass. Figures 73B and C are power and color Doppler sonograms demonstrating extrinsic compression of the splenic portal venous confluence by a rounded hypoechoic mass (arrows, Fig. 73C). The contrast-enhanced CT (Fig. 73D) confirms the nodal tissue encasing the splenoportal confluence (arrow). Figure 73E is a pathologic specimen taken from this peripancreatic node demonstrating replacement with cancer.

Diagnosis

Pancreatic carcinoma metastatic to peripancreatic lymph nodes.

Discussion

Because of its superior ability to identify liver metastasis and subtle degrees of vascular encasement, CT is generally the imaging method of choice to evaluate patients with suspected pancreatic neoplasms. With improved resolution of color and power Doppler sonography, however, even subtle peripancreatic lymph adenopathy can be detected, as in this case. Because the peripancreatic lymph node was found to be metastatic at the time of surgery, a Whipple procedure was not performed, thus sparing the patient fruitless radical surgery. Power Doppler should be used to search for arterial encasement and venous occlusion in all cases of suspected pancreatic carcinoma.

References

Bude RO, Rubin JM, Adler RS. Power versus conventional color Doppler sonography: comparison in the depiction of normal intrarenal vasculature. *Radiology* 1994;192:777–780.

Rubin JM, Bude RO, Carson PL, Bree RL, Adler RS. Power Doppler US: a potentially useful alternative to mean frequency based color Doppler US *Radiology* 1994;190:853–856.

SECTION 5

The Kidney

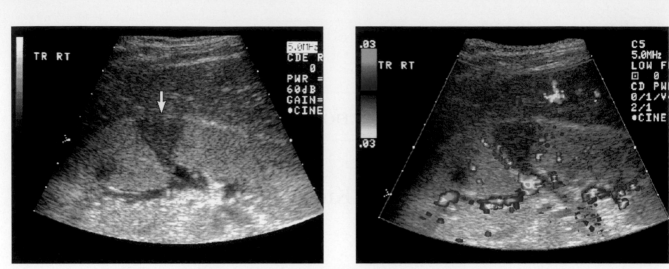

FIG. 74A. Grayscale.   FIG. 74B. Color Doppler.

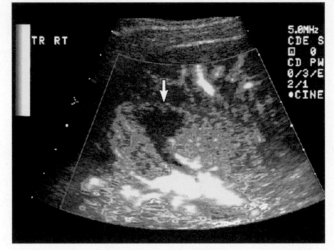

FIG. 74C. Power Doppler.

History

A 55-year-old female with acute right flank pain. Rule out renal calculus.

Findings

Figure 74A, a grayscale sonogram of the right kidney, demonstrates a peripheral wedge-shaped hypoechoic lesion in the kidney (arrow). There is increased echogenicity of the renal parenchyma. Figure 74B, a color Doppler sonogram of the right kidney, demonstrates absence of flow within this hypoechoic area. In Fig. 74C, a power Doppler sonogram, a faint area of flow is identified on the periphery of this abnormality (arrow).

Diagnosis

Acute renal infarction secondary to endocarditis.

Discussion

This patient subsequently proved to have bacterial endocarditis and underlying medical renal disease. CT (not included) confirmed multiple bilateral renal infarcts. From a morphologic standpoint, the wedge-shaped hypoechoic area in this patient strongly suggested the diagnosis of infarction. Focal pyelonephritis, however, may occasionally be confined to a single lobe and have a wedge-shaped configuration. Of note is that the power Doppler sonogram demonstrated the "cortical rim sign" that is often evident with contrast-enhanced CT. This is probably due to capsular collaterals that supply a small periphery of cortex. This finding is generally not evident in patients with pyelonephritis. The cortical rim sign was evident only on the power Doppler and was not seen with conventional color Doppler.

References

Eggli KD, Eggli D. Color Doppler sonography in pyelonephritis. *Pediatr Radiol* 1992;22:422–425.
Kass EJ, Fink-Bennett D, Cacciarelli AA, Balon H, Pavlock S. The sensitivity of renal scintigraphy and sonography in detecting nonobstructive acute pyelonephritis. *J Urol* 1992;148:606–608.

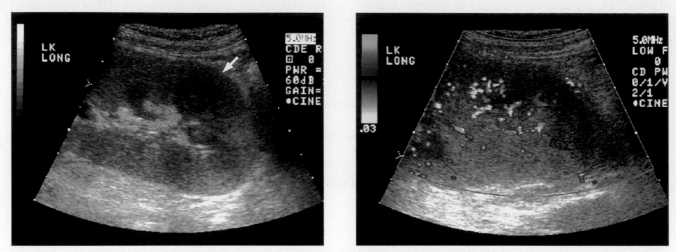

FIG. 75A. Grayscale.

FIG. 75B. Color Doppler.

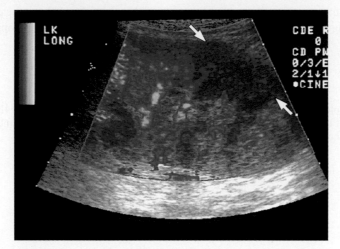

FIG. 75C. Power Doppler.

History

A 64-year-old male with sudden onset of left flank pain.

Findings

Figure 75A, a grayscale sonogram of the left kidney, demonstrates a vague hypoechoic area (arrow) in the anterior cortex of the lower pole. Figure 75B is a color Doppler sonogram demonstrating slightly decreased vascularity in the cortex in this region. Figure 75C is a power Doppler sonogram outlining a focal hypoechoic area with absent parenchymal flow (arrows).

Diagnosis

Left renal infarct.

Discussion

The differential diagnosis of the hypovascular renal abnormality in this patient includes pyelonephritis, renal abscess, infarct, or hypovascular tumor. This patient had atrial fibrillation and embolized to the left kidney and brain. The patient died of an embolic stroke and, at autopsy, multiple renal infarcts of both kidneys were identified, with a large renal infarct in the left lower pole. Power Doppler sonography was able to define the avascular area of infarction more precisely. The Doppler findings are not specific for infarction, however, as a variety of other lesions (e.g., pyelonephritis, abscess, and hypervascular tumor) can cause absent or markedly diminished flow in the renal cortex. Power Doppler is thus a sensitive but nonspecific technique for the evaluation of renal parenchymal vascular abnormalities.

References

Eggli KD, Eggli D. Color Doppler sonography in pyelonephritis. *Pediatr Radiol* 1992;22:422–425.

Kass EJ, Fink-Bennett D, Cacciarelli AA, Balon H, Pavlock S. The sensitivity of renal scintigraphy and sonography in detecting nonobstructive acute pyelonephritis. *J Urol* 1992;148:606–608.

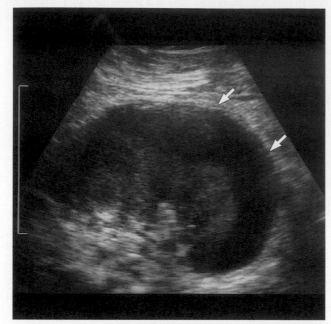

FIG. 76A. Grayscale.

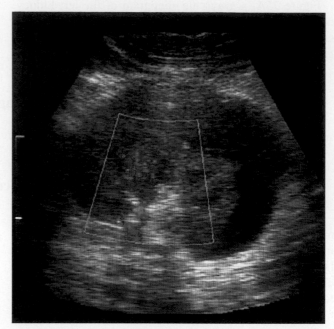

FIG. 76B. Color Doppler.

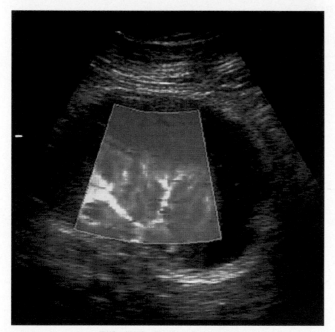

FIG. 76C. Power Doppler.

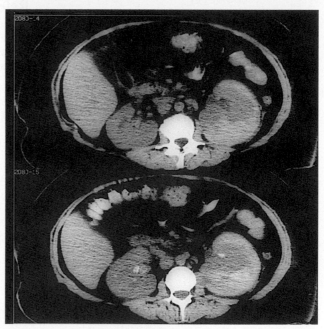

FIG. 76D. Noncontrast CT.

History

A 48-year-old female who underwent left renal biopsy because of unexplained renal failure and had acute left flank pain 1 week later.

Findings

Figure 76A is a longitudinal sonogram revealing a hypoechoic collection in the subcapsular space (arrows). The kidney is irregularly shaped and compressed, an appearance that can be confusing sonographically. Figure 76B is a color Doppler sonogram showing flow within the kidney, but not within the subcapsular collection. Figure 76C, a power Doppler sonogram in the same region, shows parenchymal flow throughout the kidney. No flow is seen, of course, in the perinephric hematoma. This clear delineation of the kidney makes the diagnosis much clearer. Figure 76D, two consecutive images from a noncontrast CT, demonstrates high-attenuation blood within the subcapsular space.

Diagnosis

Perinephric hematoma.

Discussion

Hematomas, which are common following renal biopsies, are readily detected by CT, but more difficult to image sonographically. Significant hematomas that cause symptoms requiring therapy or transfusion are rare. This patient was managed with supportive therapy and did not require narcotic analgesia or transfusion. Although the diagnosis is evident from the grayscale image, the parenchymal perfusion provided by the color Doppler and, more dramatically, by the power Doppler sonograms makes the diagnosis more readily apparent.

Reference

Ralls PW, Barakos JA, Kaptein EM, et al. Renal biopsy-related hemorrhage: frequency and comparison of CT and sonography. *J Comput Assist Tomogr* 1987;11:1031–1034.

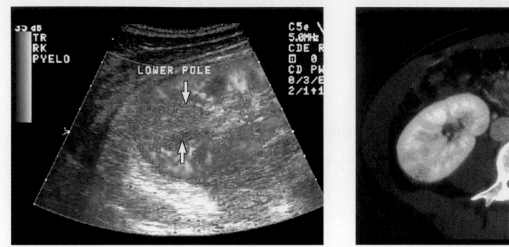

FIG. 77A. Power Doppler.

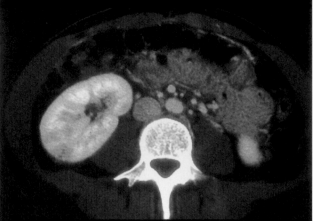

FIG. 77B. Contrast-enhanced CT.

History

A 49-year-old male with right flank pain and low-grade fever. Rule out renal calculus or obstruction.

Findings

Figure 77A is a transverse power Doppler of the lower pole of the right kidney. Note the patchy areas of decreased perfusion involving the cortex and medulla (arrows). Figure 77B is a contrast-enhanced CT scan of the right kidney. Note the focal areas of decreased contrast enhancement.

Diagnosis

Acute pyelonephritis.

Discussion

The grayscale images of this patient's right kidney were unremarkable. The ischemic areas involved with pyelonephritis were identified only with the use of power Doppler. The ability to identify very tiny cortical branches that create a cortical blush is of considerable clinical value because small areas of parenchymal ischemia can readily be detected. Pyelonephritis results in areas of decreased perfusion in the affected regions of the kidney. The reasons for this are probably multifactorial, but recently it has been noted that endotoxins from bacteria infecting the kidney activate complement. Complement aggregates then obstruct renal capillaries and cause decreased perfusion. Prior to the development of power Doppler, acute pyelonephritis could not be diagnosed reliably with either grayscale or conventional color Doppler imaging. Although the differential diagnosis includes ischemia, infarct, and hypovascular tumor, in the setting of fever and flank pain the most likely diagnosis is pyelonephritis.

References

Eggli KD, Eggli D. Color Doppler sonography in pyelonephritis. *Pediatr Radiol* 1992;22:422–425.
Kass EJ, Fink Bennett D, Cacciarelli AA, Balon H, Pavlock S. The sensitivity of renal scintigraphy and sonography in detecting nonobstructive acute pyelonephritis. *J Urol* 1992;148:606–608.

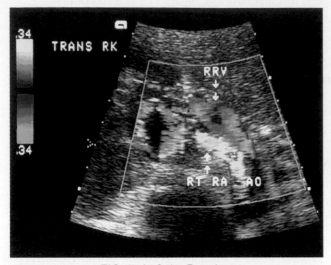

FIG. 78A. Color Doppler.

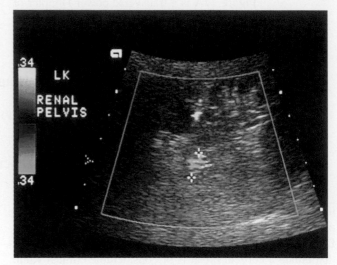

FIG. 78B. Color Doppler.

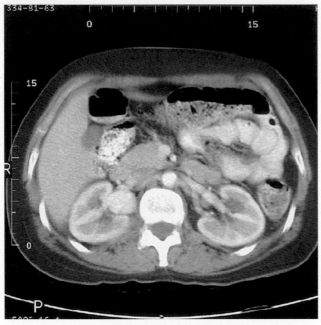

FIG. 78C. Contrast-enhanced CT.

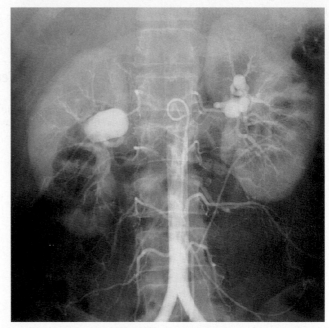

FIG. 78D. Aortogram.

History

A 22-year-old female with right flank pain who was noted to have intractable hypertension. Sonography of the right upper quadrant was ordered to evaluate the pain and to determine whether renal artery stenosis was present.

Findings

Figure 78A, a transverse color Doppler sonogram in the region of the right renal sinus, reveals a large, 2-cm renal artery aneurysm with swirling, blue- and red-coded flow within it. Figure 78B, a coronal color Doppler sonogram of the left renal pelvis, reveals a smaller, ~1-cm left-sided aneurysm that is associated with smaller tangled vessels. Figure 78C is a contrast-enhanced CT confirming the presence of the right aneurysm and the left-sided malformation. Figure 78D is an aortogram showing the large right renal artery aneurysm and a tangled aneurysmally dilated arterial mass in the left renal pelvis.

Diagnosis

Bilateral renal artery aneurysms from an unknown angiodysplasia.

Discussion

Renal artery aneurysm occurs in ~0.1% to 0.3% of the population and is an unusual cause of renal vascular hypertension. Atherosclerotic disease and fibromuscular dysplasia are more common causes. In this patient, bilateral nephrectomy with autotransplantation to the right iliac fossa was performed.

Reference

Bauer SB, Perlmutter AD, Retik AB. Anomalies of the upper urinary tract. In: Walsh PC, Retik AB, Stamey TA, Vaughan ED, eds. *Campbell's urology.* 6th ed. Philadelphia: WB Saunders, 1992:1386.

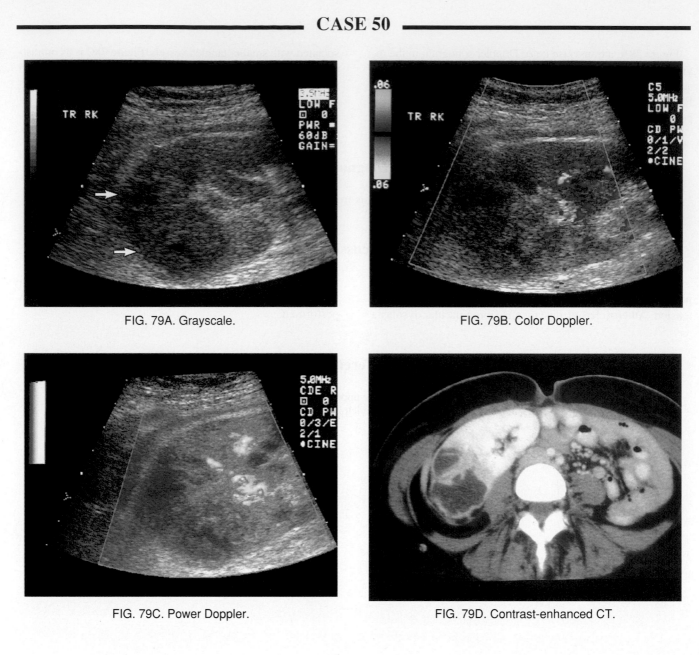

FIG. 79A. Grayscale.

FIG. 79B. Color Doppler.

FIG. 79C. Power Doppler.

FIG. 79D. Contrast-enhanced CT.

History

A 61-year-old diabetic male with a 10-day history of fever and flank pain.

Findings

Figure 79A, a grayscale transverse sonogram of the right kidney, shows a hypoechoic mass in the posterior cortex (arrows). Figure 79B, a color Doppler sonogram in the same anatomic area, demonstrates decreased perfusion to the lower pole of the right kidney. Figure 79C is a power Doppler sonogram demonstrating a large regional area of absent perfusion in the lower pole of the right kidney. Figure 79D, a contrast-enhanced CT scan performed 48 hours later, reveals a large lower-pole abscess.

Diagnosis

Right renal abscess diagnosed by power Doppler.

Discussion

The focal area of absent perfusion in the right lower pole in this patient's right kidney was caused by a renal abscess, which was successfully treated with a combination of percutaneous drainage and antibiotic therapy. The power Doppler images are nonspecific for abscess, however, because pyelonephritis, infarct, or hypovascular tumor may have a somewhat similar appearance of marked diminished perfusion. Because this patient's condition failed to respond to intravenous antibiotic therapy, a contrast-enhanced CT was performed that documented the renal abscess. It may be extremely difficult with sonography to differentiate early renal abscess formation from pyelonephritis. As the abscess enlarges, more mass effect is noted. One advantage of contrast-enhanced CT is that areas of pyelonephritis and abscess formation can be differentiated on the basis of attenuation values.

References

Eggli KD, Eggli D. Color Doppler sonography in pyelonephritis. *Pediatr Radiol* 1992;22:422–425.
Kass EJ, Fink-Bennett D, Cacciarelli AA, Balon H, Pavlock S. The sensitivity of renal scintigraphy and sonography in detecting nonobstructive acute pyelonephritis. *J Urol* 1992;148:606–608.

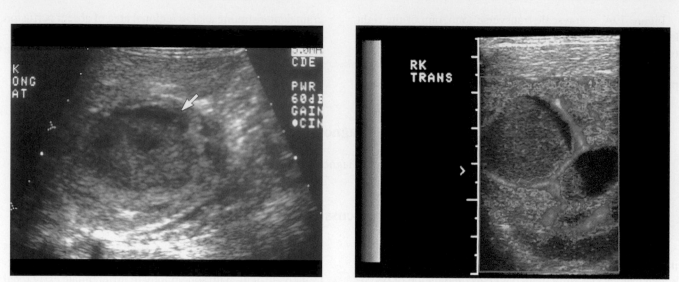

FIG. 80A. Grayscale.

FIG. 80B. Power Doppler.

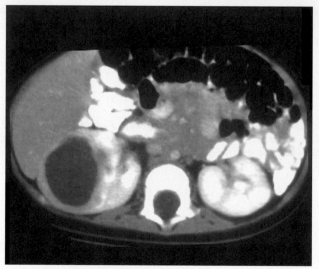

FIG. 80C. Contrast-enhanced CT.

History

A 5-year-old male with abdominal pain and febrile illness for 1 week.

Findings

Figure 80A, a sagittal sonogram of the right kidney, demonstrates an echogenic mass in the midpole (arrow). Figure 80B is a power Doppler sonogram. Note that the echogenic mass is entirely avascular. Figure 80C is a contrast-enhanced CT demonstrating a cystic mass consistent with an abscess in the kidney.

Diagnosis

Right renal abscess diagnosed with power Doppler.

Discussion

With grayscale imaging alone, the echogenic mass in this patient's kidney could have represented a neoplasm. Because it was entirely avascular with power Doppler, however, a complex cystic mass was strongly suggested. This was confirmed with a contrast-enhanced CT. This patient underwent a successful percutaneous drainage of the right renal abscess.

Note that the echogenic debris within the abscess cavity is quite apparent on the sonogram, but is difficult to appreciate on contrast-enhanced CT. The CT could be confused as showing a simple cyst. However, the clinical history and the fact that simple cysts are truly rare among children strongly suggested the diagnosis of abscess.

References

Eggli KD, Eggli D. Color Doppler sonography in pyelonephritis. *Pediatr Radiol* 1992;22:422–425.

Kass EJ, Fink-Bennett D, Cacciarelli AA, Balon H, Pavlock S. The sensitivity of renal scintigraphy and sonography in detecting nonobstructive acute pyelonephritis. *J Urol* 1992;148:606–608.

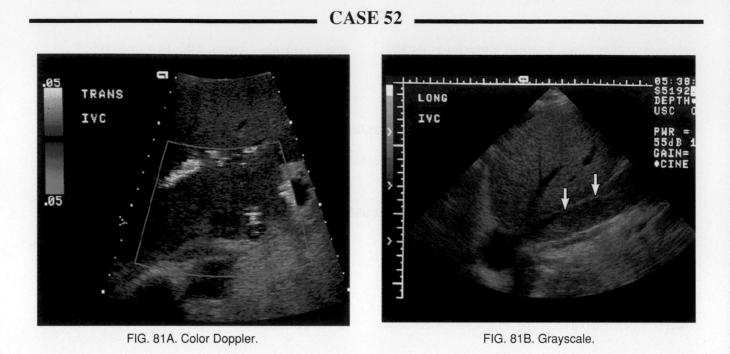

FIG. 81A. Color Doppler.

FIG. 81B. Grayscale.

History

A patient with biopsy-proven nephrotic syndrome who had syncope. Pulmonary embolism was suspected and a study was requested to evaluate the renal veins and inferior vena cava.

Findings

Figure 81A, a transverse color Doppler sonogram of the inferior vena cava, demonstrates nearly total thrombosis of the inferior vena cava filled with a moderately echogenic clot.

Figure 81B, a longitudinal sonogram of the inferior vena cava, shows a large clot extending to the level of the hepatic veins tapering cephalically.

Diagnosis

Nephrotic syndrome with inferior vena caval clot.

Discussion

Nephrotic syndrome is a condition characterized by heavy proteinuria, hypoalbuminuria, hyperlipidemia and lipiduria, and edema. Because of the pronounced changes in protein balance that occur, blood levels of many clotting and anticoagulant factors are abnormally decreased or increased in nephrotic syndrome. Thus, hypercoagulation with venous and arterial thrombosis may occur. Likewise, abnormal bleeding may result. Most patients with nephrotic syndrome have no venous thrombosis. Prevalence varies from 2% to 28% for renal vein clot. Thrombus is often found in patients with membranous or membranoproliferative glomeru-lonephritis. Minimal-change-disease nephritis and other conditions that cause nephrotic syndrome occasionally have associated venous clot. It is debated whether primary thrombus causes nephrotic syndrome. Most nephrologists feel that the nephrotic syndrome, because of hypercoagulability, causes thrombosis. Most patients with thrombosis related to nephrotic syndrome have thrombus isolated in the renal veins. Occasionally, inferior vena caval clots may occur, such as in this case. Pulmonary embolism is a well-known complication of nephrotic syndrome. It seems reasonable to assume that inferior vena caval clot has a higher risk of this complication.

Reference

Massry SG, Vaziri ND. Glomerular diseases: thromboembolic complications. In: *Massry and Glassock's textbook of nephrology*. 3rd ed. Baltimore: Williams and Wilkins, 1995:690–694.

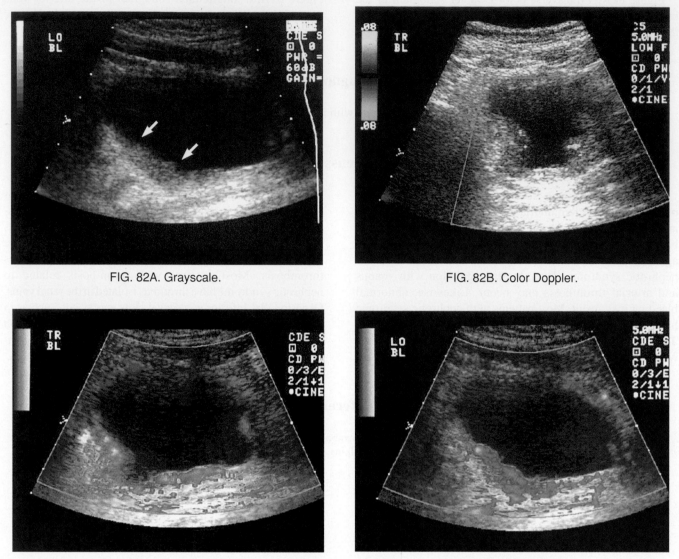

FIG. 82A. Grayscale.

FIG. 82B. Color Doppler.

FIG. 82C. Power Doppler.

FIG. 82D. Power Doppler.

History

A 42-year-old female with hematuria and dysuria following chemotherapy for Wegener's granulomatosis of the lung.

Findings

Figure 82A, a grayscale image of the bladder, demonstrates thickening of the posterior bladder wall (arrows). Figure 82B, a transverse color Doppler sonogram of the bladder, shows focally increased mural vascularity. On power Doppler (Figs. 82C and D), however, marked hyperemia of the entire bladder wall is noted.

Diagnosis

Cytoxan cystitis diagnosed with power Doppler.

Discussion

The power Doppler images in this case strongly suggested an inflammatory process involving the entire bladder wall. A history of Cytoxan (cyclophosphamide) administration for Wegener's granulomatosis suggested a diagnosis of Cytoxan cystitis. The patient's symptoms markedly improved following cessation of chemotherapy. Cystoscopic biopsies revealed nonspecific inflammation without evidence of tumor. Although the mural thickening identified with grayscale imaging was suggestive of cystitis, the power Doppler was more useful in this case in demonstrating the significantly increased flow in this lesion.

Reference

Day DL, Carpenter BL. Abdominal complications in pediatric bone marrow transplant recipients. *Radiographics* 1993;13:1101–1112.

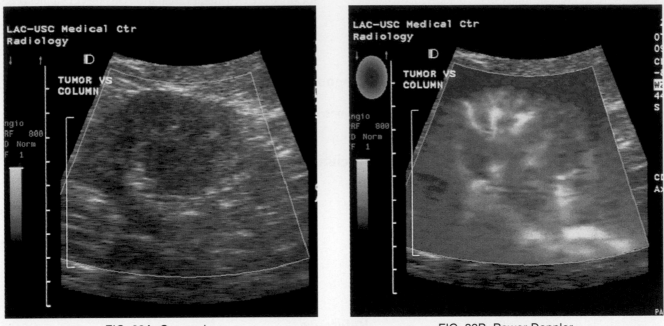

FIG. 83A. Grayscale.

FIG. 83B. Power Doppler.

History

A 52-year-old male with left flank pain and microhematuria whose intravenous pyelogram revealed a questionable renal sinus mass. Ultrasound was recommended.

Findings

Figure 83A is a grayscale sonogram showing a possible renal sinus mass in the upper pole of the left kidney. Figure 83B is a power Doppler angiogram revealing that this mass is equivalent in its blood flow to surrounding portions of the kidney.

Diagnosis

The renal column simulated renal cell carcinoma.

Discussion

Although the color flow pattern of renal cell carcinoma has not been fully elucidated, our experience is that normal flow is incompatible with the diagnosis of neoplasm. Thus, other examinations such as CT scan or radionuclide imaging are unnecessary in this patient.

References

Bude RO, Rubin JM, Adler RS. Power versus conventional color Doppler sonography: comparison in the depiction of normal intrarenal vasculature. *Radiology* 1994;192:777–780.

Rubin JM, Bude RO, Carson PL, et al. Power Doppler US: potentially useful alternative to mean frequency based color Doppler US. *Radiology* 1994;190:853–856.

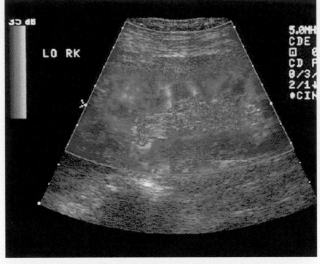

FIG. 84A. Power Doppler.

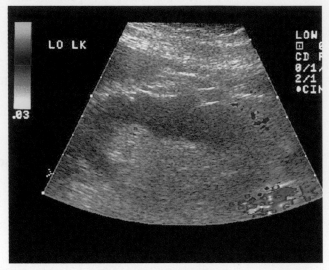

FIG. 84B. Color Doppler.

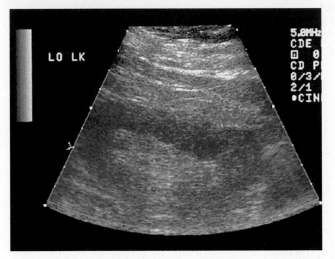

FIG. 84C. Power Doppler.

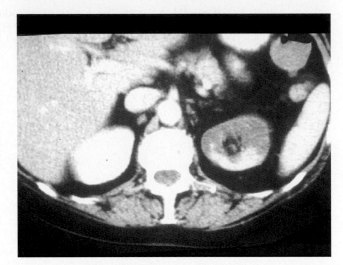

FIG. 84D. Contrast-enhanced CT.

History

A 63-year-old female with acute left flank pain. Rule out hydronephrosis or obstruction.

Findings

Figure 84A, a normal power Doppler of the right kidney, shows a symmetric cortical blush. Figure 84B, a color Doppler sonogram of the left kidney, demonstrates markedly diminished flow to the kidney. Figure 84C is a power Doppler also confirming these findings. Figure 84D is a contrast-enhanced CT demonstrating extensive areas of infarction in the left kidney.

Diagnosis

Left renal infarction.

Discussion

This patient's embolic infarct to the left kidney was caused by a left ventricular thrombus. The patient was in atrial fibrillation and had not been taking her oral anticoagulants. Both color and power Doppler demonstrated almost complete absence of flow to the left kidney consistent with an infarct. This was confirmed on a subsequent contrast-enhanced CT. The grayscale images of the kidney alone are relatively unremarkable, and thus color and power Doppler should be used routinely in any patient who has an acute renal process such as pyelonephritis, abscess, or infarct.

References

Bude RO, Rubin JM, Adler RS. Power versus conventional color Doppler sonography: comparison in the depiction of normal intrarenal vasculature. *Radiology* 1994;192:777–780.

Newman JS, Adler RS, Bude RO, Rubin JM. Detection of soft-tissue hyperemia: value of power Doppler sonography. *AJR* 1994;163:385–389.

Rubin JM, Bude RO, Carson PL, et al. Power Doppler US: a potentially useful alternative to mean frequency based color Doppler US. *Radiology* 1994;190:853–856.

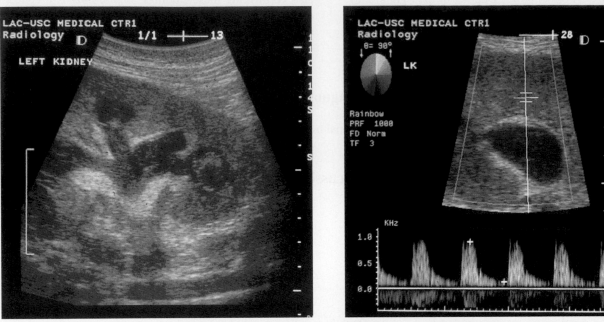

FIG. 85A. Grayscale.

FIG. 85B. Doppler spectrum.

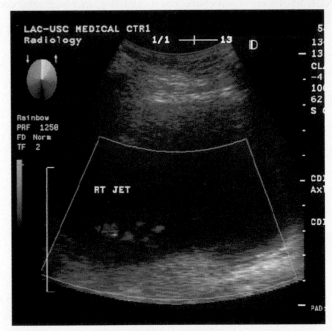

FIG. 85C. Color Doppler.

History

A 38-year-old diabetic female with fever and left flank pain. Because of poor renal function, a sonogram was ordered.

Findings

Figure 85A, a longitudinal sonogram of the left kidney, reveals moderate hydronephrosis with a castlike filling defect in most of the intrarenal collecting system. Figure 85B is a color Doppler guided spectral sonogram revealing elevated peripheral resistance in the intrarenal arterial branches (resistive index = 0.84; normal = 0.70). Figure 85C, a color Doppler sonogram through the bladder, shows a right ureteral jet. No left ureteral jet was identified during 10 minutes of observation.

Diagnosis

Pyonephrosis.

Discussion

Hydronephrosis and debris in the setting of potential infection in a diabetic patient should strongly suggest the diagnosis of pyonephrosis. Unfortunately, internal debris within the collecting system is seen in only approximately half of patients with pyonephrosis. A strong clinical suspicion of pyonephrosis should prompt percutaneous nephrostomy. Two Doppler signs of ureteral obstruction were present in this patient. The abnormally high intrarenal artery peripheral resistance, manifest as an elevated resistive index, strongly suggested the diagnosis of obstruction. The absent left ureteral jet after 10 minutes of observation when right-sided ureteral jets were present was virtually diagnostic of obstruction.

Reference

Jeffrey RB Jr, Ralls PW. The kidney and adrenal gland. In: *CT and sonography of the acute abdomen.* 2nd ed. Philadelphia: Lippincott–Raven, 1996:224–228.

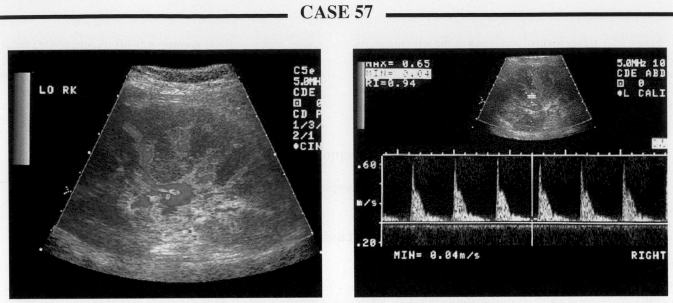

FIG. 86A. Power Doppler.

FIG. 86B. Doppler spectrum.

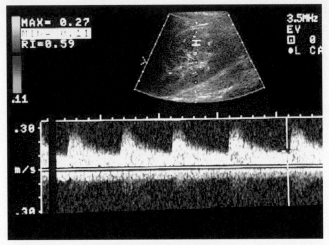

FIG. 86C. Doppler spectrum.

History

A 26-year-old female with bipolar disorder (manic depression) who had bilateral flank pain, hematuria, and a markedly elevated serum creatinine level.

Findings

Figure 86A, a power Doppler sonogram of the right kidney, demonstrates marked pruning of the intrarenal vasculature. A similar appearance was noted in the left kidney (not shown). Figure 86B, a spectral Doppler tracing from the right kidney, demonstrates significantly dampened diastolic flow with a high resistive index. Figure 86C, a follow-up Doppler spectrum 3 weeks later following cessation of lithium therapy, demonstrates normal renal flow.

Diagnosis

Interstitial nephritis secondary to lithium toxicity.

Discussion

The power Doppler sonogram in this case demonstrated marked pruning of renal parenchymal vascularity bilaterally with a high resistive index consistent with acute medical renal disease. The high doses of lithium that the patient had been taking for bipolar disorder resulted in acute interstitial nephritis. Following the withdrawal of the medication, the patient's diastolic flow normalized. Note the normal resistive index in Fig. 86C. This case illustrates the value of power Doppler imaging of the renal vasculature. The grayscale images were essentially normal. The bilaterally symmetric pruning of the parenchymal vasculature strongly suggested medical renal disease as the cause of the patient's acute renal insufficiency. The patient's creatinine level also returned to normal.

References

Helenon O, Attlan E, Legendre C, et al. Gd-DOTA-enhanced MR imaging and color Doppler US of renal allograft necrosis. *Radiographics* 1992;12:21–33.

Kass EJ, Fink-Bennett D, Cacciarelli AA, Balon H, Pavlock S. The sensitivity of renal scintigraphy and sonography in detecting nonobstructive acute pyelonephritis. *J Urol* 1992;148:606–608.

Walker RG. Lithium nephrotoxicity. *Kidney Int Suppl* 1993;42:S93–S98.

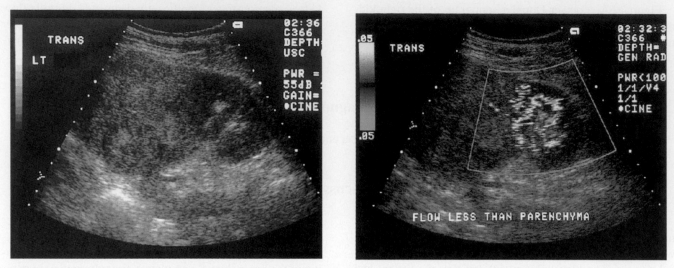

FIG. 87A. Patient 1.   FIG. 87B. Patient 1.

History

Seven different patients.

148

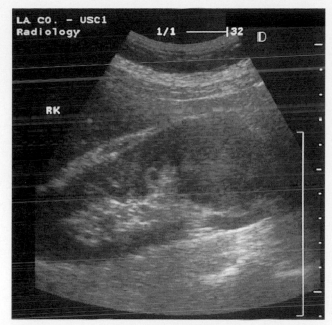

FIG. 87C. Patient 2.

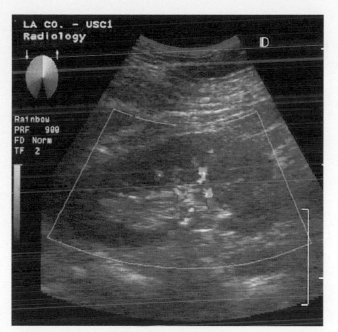

FIG. 87D. Patient 2.

Findings

Figure 87A is a grayscale image showing a large upper-pole left-sided renal cell carcinoma. Figure 87B is a color Doppler sonogram demonstrating markedly decreased flow in this renal cell carcinoma. Flow is much less than in the normal renal cortex. Figure 87C shows another case, in which a moderate-sized lower-pole right-sided renal cell carcinoma is identified. Figure 87D demonstrates that this lesion, too, has less flow than does normal renal parenchyma. A small amount of internal flow is noted in the caudal aspect of the lesion. Figure 87E shows a large right-sided renal cell carcinoma exhibiting no internal flow. Prominent peripheral flow is imaged. Flow in the renal cell carcinoma is less than in the contiguous renal cortex. Figure 87F shows a small left-sided renal cell carcinoma exhibiting greater flow than contiguous renal cortex. Figure 87G demonstrates another small left-sided renal cell carcinoma exhibiting increased flow compared with the renal cortex. Figure 87H, a grayscale image of the same case, shows the mixed echogenicity of the lesion. There is considerable morphologic distortion with impingement on the renal sinus, as well as exophytic growth outside the normal renal contours. Figure 87I shows a left-sided renal cell carcinoma with increased flow, primarily peripheral. Figure 87J demonstrates a calcified right-sided renal cell carcinoma exhibiting prominent peripheral and internal flow, much greater than that of the contiguous renal cortex.

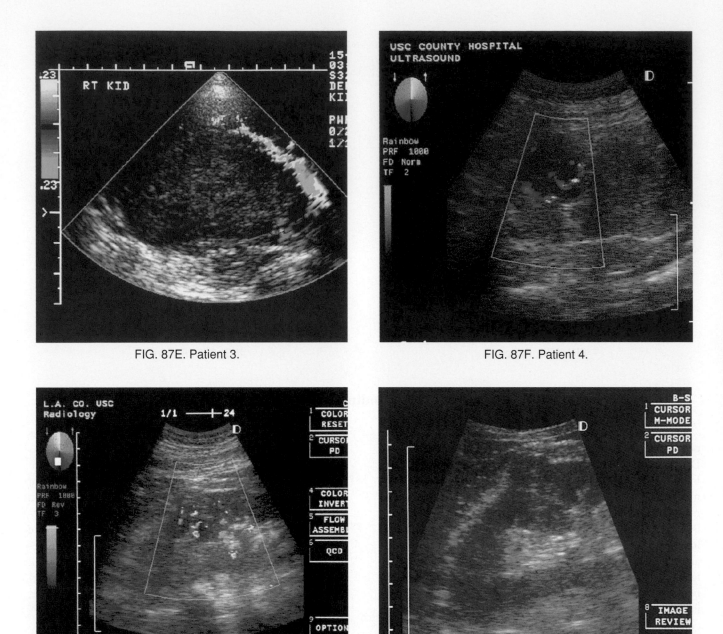

FIG. 87E. Patient 3.

FIG. 87F. Patient 4.

FIG. 87G. Patient 5.

FIG. 87H. Patient 5.

Diagnosis

Blood flow in several different renal cell carcinomas.

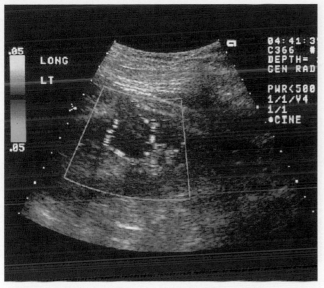

FIG. 87I. Patient 6.

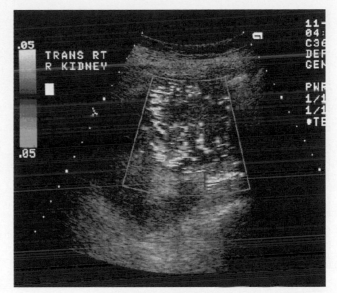

FIG. 87J. Patient 7.

Discussion

Although the exact characteristics of color Doppler flow in renal cell carcinomas are currently incompletely described, most renal cell carcinomas seem to have less internal flow than does the adjacent renal cortex. This is distinct from angiography, where ≥75% of renal cell carcinomas are hypervascular. Although the reasons for this difference are unclear, angiography may show slowly flowing blood that pools within and around the lesion. The Doppler shift of slowly flowing blood may be insufficient to be detected routinely by color flow imaging. Although the degree of flow within renal cell carcinomas is variable, we have yet to encounter a renal cell carcinoma with normal flow patterns similar to that of normal renal parenchyma. For this reason, we feel that the presence of normal renal flow on color flow imaging virtually eliminates the possibility of a renal cell carcinoma.

References

Hirai T, Ohishi H, Yamada R, et al. Usefulness of color Doppler flow imaging in differential diagnosis of multilocular cystic lesions of the kidney. *J Ultrasound Med* 1995;14:771–776.

Kier R, Taylor KJW, Feyock AL, et al. Renal masses: characterization with Doppler US. *Radiology* 1990; 176:703–707.

Kuijpers D, Jaspers R. Renal mass: differential diagnosis with pulsed Doppler US. *Radiology* 1989,170:59–60.

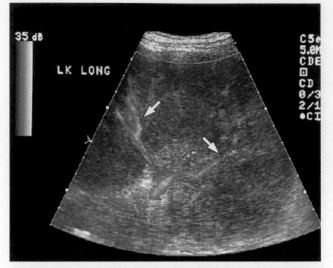

FIG. 88A. Power Doppler.

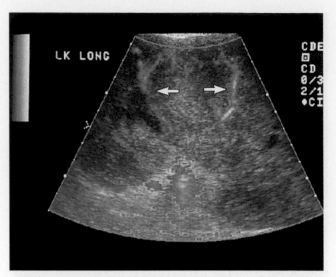

FIG. 88B. Power Doppler.

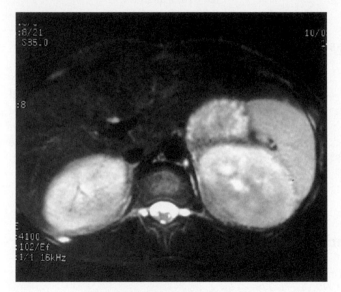

FIG. 88C. MRI with gadolinium.

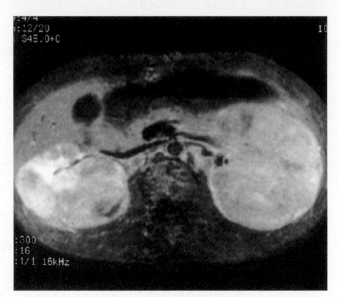

FIG. 88D. MRI with gadolinium.

History

A 9-year-old female with back pain and rising creatinine level.

Findings

Figures 88A and B are power Doppler sonograms of the left kidney that demonstrate marked splaying of the intrarenal vasculature (arrows). Large hypoechoic masses are noted replacing much of the kidney. Similar masses were noted in the right kidney. Figures 88C and D are gadolinium-enhanced MRIs demonstrating bilateral renal masses.

Diagnosis

Non-Hodgkin's lymphoma of the kidneys.

Discussion

The power Doppler images in this case were quite useful to demonstrate vascular displacement by multiple hypovascular masses. The vascular splaying is consistent with mass effect. Diagnostic considerations in a patient with focal areas of hypoperfusion include pyelonephritis and infarction. Neither of these two lesions, however, is associated with significant mass effect. Evolution of an area of pyelonephritis into an abscess, however, will be accompanied by significant mass effect, although the grayscale image should demonstrate features of a complex cystic mass. In the differential diagnosis of bilateral hypoechoic renal masses, lymphoma must always be considered. Renal lymphoma is almost always non-Hodgkin's lymphoma. It is not unusual to have renal involvement in patient's with AIDS-related lymphomas. There may be relatively little, if any, associated nodal involvement.

References

Eisenberg PJ, Papanicolaou N, Lee MJ, Yoder IC. Diagnostic imaging in the evaluation of renal lymphoma. *Leuk Lymphoma* 1994;16:37–50.

Weinberger E, Rosenbaum DM, Pendergrass TW. Renal involvement in children with lymphoma: comparison of CT with sonography. *AJR* 1990;155:347–349.

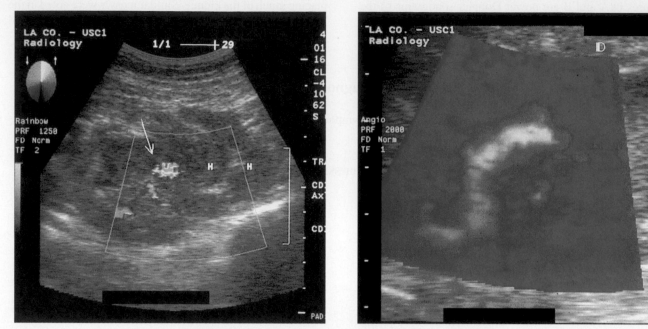

FIG. 89A. Color Doppler.

FIG. 89B. Power Doppler.

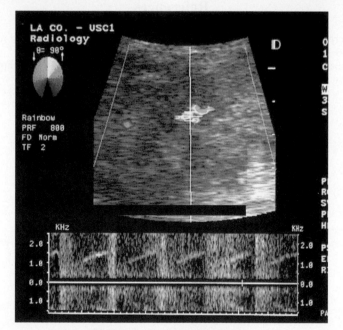

FIG. 89C. Doppler spectrum.

History

After renal biopsy, a patient with local pain around the biopsy site, a five-point drop in hematocrit, and hematuria. Renal sonography was ordered.

154

Findings

Figure 89A is a color Doppler sonogram showing a focal collection of blood flow with high-velocity aliased flow. Figure 89B is a magnified power Doppler image demonstrating similar findings, but a prominent vessel leading toward the abnormal flow area is noted. Figure 89C, spectral Doppler in the abnormal area, reveals very turbulent high-velocity flow.

Diagnosis

Post-renal-biopsy arteriovenous fistula.

Discussion

Acquired arteriovenous fistula accounts for 75% of all renal arteriovenous fistulas. Arteriovenous fistula subsequent to renal biopsy is the most common cause. Most are asymptomatic. This patient was symptomatic because of hemorrhage associated with the fistula and biopsy. The lesion was successfully diagnosed based on the enlarged vascular space within the kidney near the site of the biopsy with turbulent flow within it. Almost all post-renal-biopsy arteriovenous fistulas, such as this one, resolve spontaneously without intervention. A follow-up color Doppler sonogram 1 week later (not shown) revealed no sign of this postbiopsy vascular malformation.

Reference

Libertino JA. Renovascular surgery. In: Walsh PC, Retik AB, Stamey TA, Vaughan ED, eds. *Campbell's urology*. 6th ed. Philadelphia: WB Saunders, 1992:2524–2525.

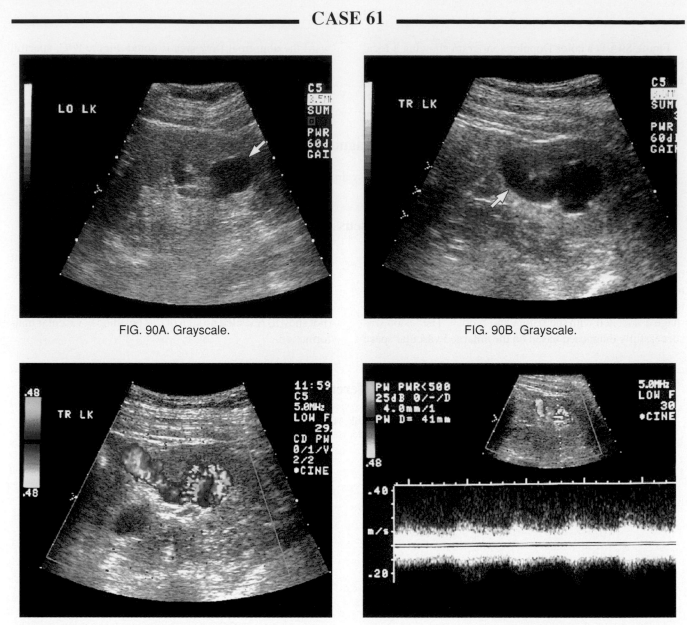

FIG. 90A. Grayscale.

FIG. 90B. Grayscale.

FIG. 90C. Color Doppler.

FIG. 90D. Doppler spectrum.

History

A 61-year-old female with a left lower-pole renal "cyst" noted on an outside sonogram.

Findings

Figures 90A and B are sagittal images of the left kidney that demonstrate a cystic mass in the lower pole (arrow, Fig. 90A). Note an adjacent tubular structure along the anterior and superior aspects of the mass in Fig. 90B (arrow). Figure 90C is a color Doppler sonogram demonstrating that the "cystic mass" represents a vascular structure adjacent to a large feeding artery. Figure 90D is spectral Doppler demonstrating pulsatile venous flow diagnostic of an arteriovenous fistula.

Diagnosis

Arteriovenous fistula of the lower pole of the kidney.

Discussion

Renal arteriovenous fistulas are most often the sequela of renal biopsy or penetrating trauma. In this case, the etiology was unknown, but may have been related to subclinical trauma. The hallmark of an arteriovenous fistula is an enlarged feeding artery, adjacent soft tissue turbulence (bruit), and pulsatile venous outflow from the fistula. As with other "cystic masses" that turn out to be vascular structures, it is always essential to keep this potential pitfall in mind and to use color Doppler to evaluate all "cystic lesions" in the abdomen. Based on the outside grayscale image, this lesion was misinterpreted as a simple cyst. This patient underwent a successful transcatheter embolization of the arteriovenous fistula without sequela

References

Crotty KL, Orihuela E, Warren MM. Recent advances in the diagnosis and treatment of renal arteriovenous malformations and fistulas. *J Urol* 1993;150:1135–1139.

Duda SH, Erley CM, Wakat JP, et al. Posttransplant renal artery stenosis: outpatient intraarterial DSA versus color aided duplex Doppler sonography. *Eur J Radiol* 1993;16:95–101.

Plainfosse MC, Calonge VM, Beyloune-Mainardi C, Glotz D, Duboust A. Vascular complications in the adult kidney transplant recipient. *J Clin Ultrasound* 1992;20:517–527.

Takebayashi S, Aida N, Matsui K. Arteriovenous malformations of the kidneys: diagnosis and follow-up with color Doppler sonography in six patients. *AJR* 1991;157:991–995.

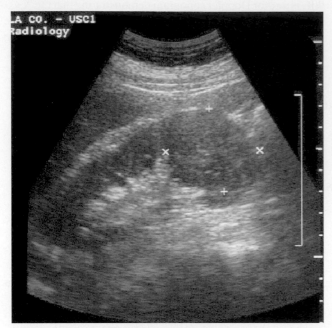

FIG. 91A. Grayscale.

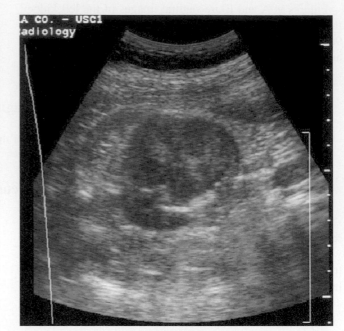

FIG. 91B. Grayscale.

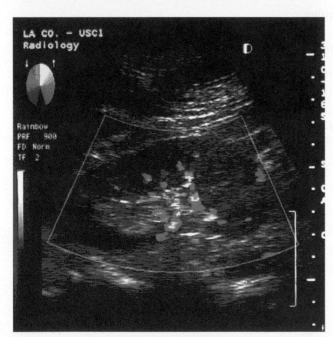

FIG. 91C. Color Doppler.

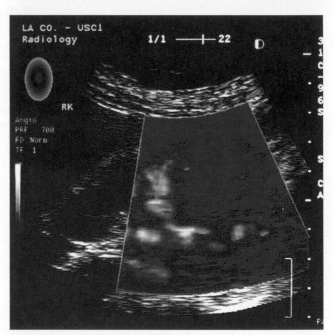

FIG. 91D. Power Doppler.

History

A 41-year-old female with right upper-quadrant pain who was referred to ultrasound for evaluation of the gallbladder for the possibility of cholelithiasis. All laboratory findings, including urinalysis, were normal.

Findings

Figures 91A and B are longitudinal and transverse real-time sonograms showing a 4-cm mass that is mixed in echogenicity compared with the renal cortex. Figure 91C is a longitudinal color Doppler sonogram revealing more flow in the normal kidney than within the mass. Only a small amount of peripheral flow is seen associated with this tumor.

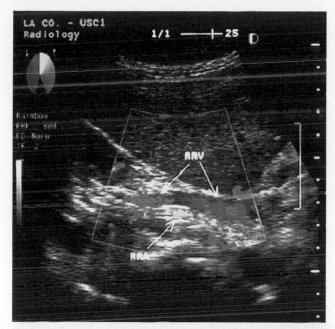

FIG. 91E. Color Doppler.

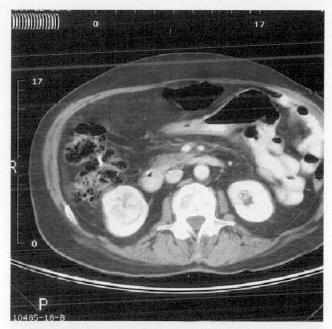

FIG. 91F. Contrast-enhanced CT.

Figure 91D is power Doppler that reveals similar findings—that is, less flow in the renal cell carcinoma than in normal renal parenchyma. Figure 91E is an oblique color Doppler sonogram of the right renal vein. Usually, the right renal vein arises from the renal hilus and courses cephalad to enter the inferior vena cava. Oblique images are therefore necessary to show its full length. No venous invasion is detected in this study. Note the right renal artery behind (dorsal to) the right renal vein. Figure 91F is a contrast-enhanced CT showing the region of the lower pole. Notice that it enhances inhomogeneously compared with the adjacent renal cortex. CT revealed renal vein invasion, lymphadenopathy, or metastatic disease.

Diagnosis

Stage-I renal cell carcinoma.

Discussion

This unsuspected finding was discovered on an upper abdominal survey performed as part of a right upper-quadrant ultrasound. It is not unusual to detect an incidental renal cell carcinoma on a right upper-quadrant or other abdominal ultrasound. Important features to seek once the mass has been discovered are venous invasion, collateral vessels, lymph nodes, and metastasis. The relatively decreased flow of the renal cell cancer compared with the normal kidney on color and power Doppler is not unusual in our experience. It is our impression (although no data exist to support this) that renal cell carcinomas are often less vascular appearing than normal kidney on color flow imaging techniques. This is distinct from findings with angiography, where 75% of renal cell carcinomas are hypervascular and only 9% are avascular. Evaluation of the renal vein is important because it affects the stage of the neoplasm and operative management. To obtain an accurate assessment of venous invasion, color Doppler is used to identify the entire length of the renal vein. This is much more difficult, or even impossible, without the use of color flow imaging. Once the vein has been identified, it should be evaluated both with and without color flow to look for clot and collateral vessels. The non-color-flow evaluation of the vein is important because color flow may occasionally overwrite a partial venous thrombosis. CT, and sometimes MRI, are performed in patients with renal cell cancer to determine the extent of disease. CT is generally more reliable than sonography in detecting nodal and other metastases. In this instance, the imaging diagnosis of a stage-I renal cell carcinoma (confined to the capsule with no venous invasion and no metastasis) was confirmed surgically.

References

Charboneau JW, Hattery RR, Ernst EC III, et al. Spectrum of sonographic findings in 125 renal masses other than benign simple cyst. *AJR* 1983;140:87–94.

Curry NS, Schabel SI, Betsill WL Jr. Small renal neoplasms: diagnostic imaging, pathologic features, and clinical course. *Radiology* 1986;158:113–117.

Levine E, Huntrakoon M, Wetzel LH. Small renal neoplasms: clinical, pathologic, and imaging features. *AJR* 1989; 153:69–73.

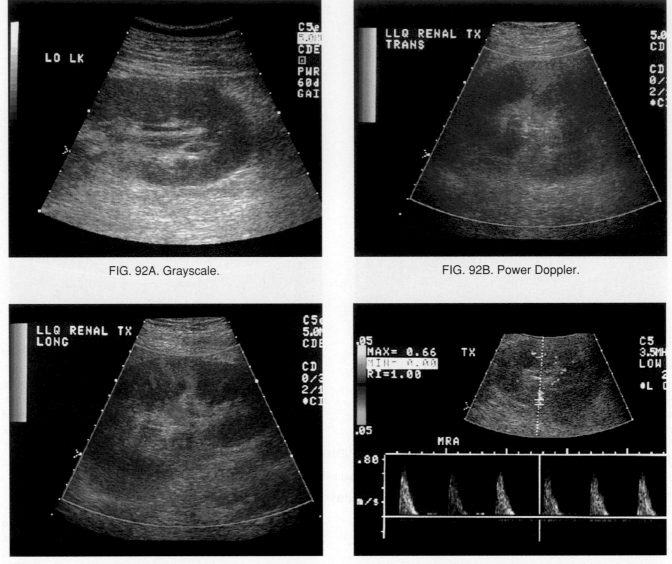

FIG. 92A. Grayscale.

FIG. 92B. Power Doppler.

FIG. 92C. Power Doppler.

FIG. 92D. Doppler spectrum.

History

Rising creatinine and anuria 48 hours after renal transplantation.

Findings

Figure 92A, a grayscale image of the renal transplant, demonstrates no evidence of hydronephrosis or other structural abnormalities. Figures 92B and C are power Doppler images of the transplanted kidney that demonstrate marked pruning of intrarenal vasculature. Figure 92D is spectral Doppler demonstrating high-resistance flow.

Diagnosis

Acute vascular rejection following renal transplantation.

Discussion

In the immediate posttransplantation period, causes of rising creatinine and anuria include acute renal obstruction, acute vascular rejection, acute tubular necrosis, and vascular occlusion of the graft. The power Doppler images clearly demonstrated that arterial flow was preserved to portions of the kidney, but that there were large ischemic areas throughout much of the renal parenchyma. However, the presence of arterial flow excluded global infarction (due to occlusion of the arterial anastamosis) as the cause of this patient's symptoms. Renal biopsy revealed acute vascular rejection of the kidney, which was aggressively treated with drug therapy. The kidney did not ultimately respond to therapy, however, and the patient required retransplantation.

References

Plainfosse MC, Calonge VM, Beyloune-Mainardi C, Glotz D, Duboust A. Vascular complications in the adult kidney transplant recipient. *J Clin Ultrasound* 1992;20:517–527.

Tublin ME, Dodd GD III. Sonography of renal transplantation. *Radiol Clin North Am* 1995;33:447–459.

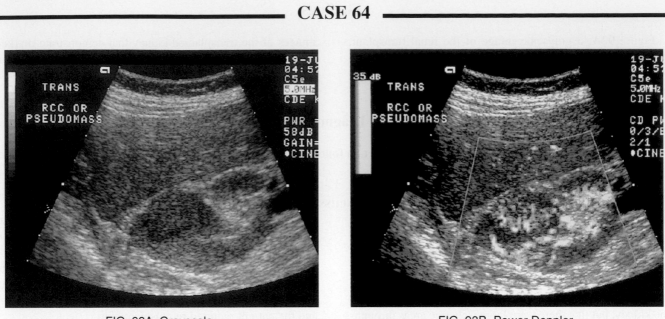

FIG. 93A. Grayscale.

FIG. 93B. Power Doppler.

History

A 57-year-old female with mild right flank pain whose urinalysis revealed microhematuria. Intravenous pyelography suggested a renal mass.

Findings

Figure 93A, a grayscale sonogram through the right kidney, reveals irregularity of the upper pole of the kidney. Figure 93B is power Doppler revealing normal flow throughout this region.

Diagnosis

Renal scar simulates renal cell carcinoma.

Discussion

Although the color flow sonographic pattern in renal cell carcinoma has not been definitively described, all renal cell carcinomas that we have seen have had flow patterns different from the normal parenchymal pattern. The normal flow shown in the power Doppler image strongly suggested that the contour irregularity did not represent a renal cell carcinoma, but rather a pseudomass, perhaps from scarring. Results of clinical follow-up were benign; eventually, a follow-up CT scan revealed no abnormality.

References

Bude RO, Rubin JM, Adler RS. Power versus conventional color Doppler sonography: comparison in the depiction of normal intrarenal vasculature. *Radiology* 1994;192:777–780.

Rubin JM, Bude RO, Carson PL, et al. Power Doppler US: potentially useful alternative to mean frequency based color Doppler US. *Radiology* 1994;190:853–856.

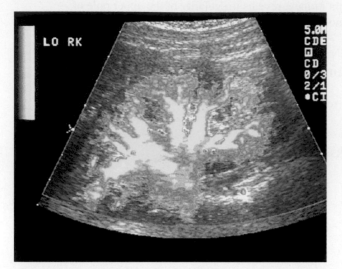

FIG. 94A. Power Doppler.

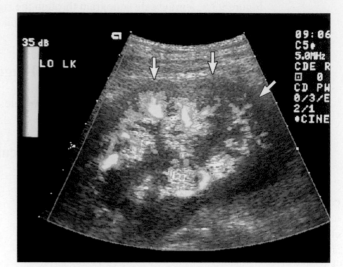

FIG. 94B. Power Doppler.

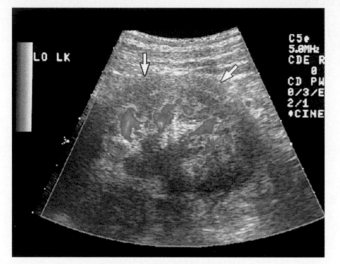

FIG. 94C. Power Doppler.

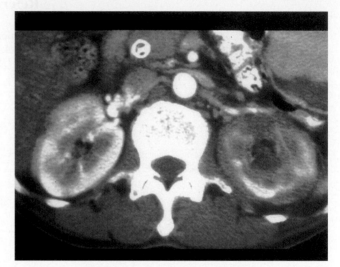

FIG. 94D. Contrast-enhanced CT.

History

Vague left flank pain. Rule out hydronephrosis.

Findings

Figure 94A, a sagittal power Doppler sonogram of the right kidney, demonstrates normal cortical flow. Figures 94B and C are power Doppler sonograms of the left kidney that demonstrate a peripheral hypoechoic mantle (arrows) of tissue that suggests cortical ischemia. Figure 94D is a contrast-enhanced CT demonstrating normal enhancement of the right renal cortex, but patchy perfusion to the cortex of the left kidney, with a low-attenuation mantle of tissue around the left kidney. Incidentally noted is a metallic stent in the common bile duct.

Diagnosis

Retroperitoneal fibrosis encasing the left kidney.

Discussion

The poor perfusion to the left kidney in this case was caused by fibrotic tissue surrounding the left kidney. At surgical exploration, the ureter was free of involvement, but the perirenal space was extensively encased by a fibrotic mass. The periaortic areas were relatively spared. Perirenal involvement is a rare manifestation of retroperitoneal fibrosis, which typically involves the periaortic area symmetrically and frequently obstructs both ureters. The power Doppler images in this case demonstrated the asymmetric cortical perfusion caused by the perirenal fibrosis. Because this is such a rare entity, however, it would be difficult to make a specific diagnosis from these images.

References

Amis ES Jr. Retroperitoneal fibrosis. *AJR* 1991;157:321–329.
Rominger MB, Kenney PJ. Perirenal involvement by retroperitoneal fibrosis: the usefulness of MRI to establish diagnosis. *Urol Radiol* 1992;13:173–176.

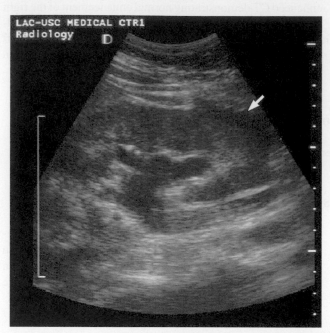

FIG. 95A. Grayscale.

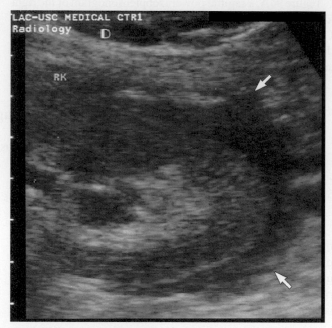

FIG. 95B. Grayscale.

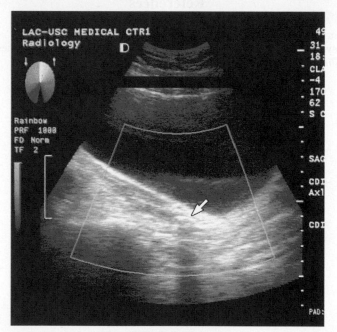

FIG. 95C. Color Doppler.

History

A 38-year-old female with excruciating right upper-quadrant and right flank pain who was afebrile and had a white count of 12,000.

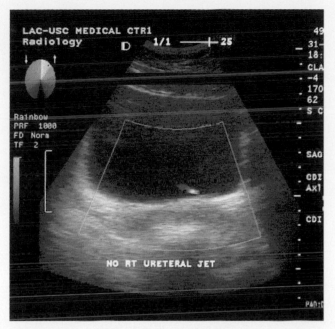

FIG. 95D. Color Doppler.

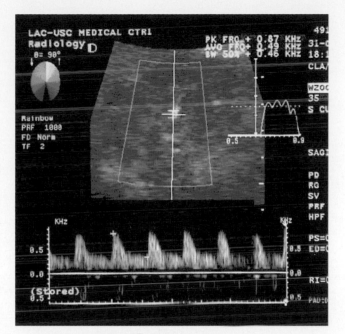

FIG. 95E. Doppler spectrum.

Findings

Figure 95A is a sagittal sonogram of the right kidney. Note the right-sided hydronephrosis and perinephric fluid (arrow). Figure 95B, a sagittal scan of the lower pole of the right kidney, shows perinephric fluid (arrows). Figure 95C is a sonogram revealing a distal right ureteral calculus (arrow). Figure 95D, a transverse sonogram of the bladder, shows a left ureteral jet, but no right ureteral jet. No jet was seen during 5 minutes of observation. Figure 95E is a color Doppler-guided spectral Doppler revealing that there is a normal resistive index in the right kidney (RI < 0.70).

Diagnosis

Forniceal rupture from distal ureteral stone.

Discussion

This is an example of perirenal extravasation related to forniceal rupture from an obstructing distal right ureteral calculus. Doppler sonography can be helpful in assessing renal obstruction in several ways. Most important in this patient is the absence of a right-sided ureteral jet, which indicates obstruction of the right distal ureter. Although many patients with acute obstruction have elevated peripheral resistance, manifest as an increased RI (>0.70) the normal RI in this patient suggests that the obstruction has been "relieved" by the forniceal rupture.

References

Baker SM, Middleton WD. Color Doppler sonography of ureteral jets in normal volunteers: importance of the relative specific gravity of urine in the ureter and bladder. *AJR* 1992;159:773–775.

Burge HJ, Middleton WD, McClennan BL, et al. Ureteral jets in healthy subjects and in patients with unilateral ureteral calculi: comparison with color Doppler US. *Radiology* 1991;180:437–442.

Deyoe LA, Cronin JJ, Breslaw BH, et al. New technologies of ultrasound and color Doppler in the prospective evaluation of acute renal obstruction: do they replace the intravenous urogram? *Abdom Imag* 1995;20:158–163.

Price CI, Adler RS, Rubin JM. Ultrasound detection of differences in density: explanation of the ureteric jet phenomenon and implications for new ultrasound applications. *Invest Radiol* 1989;24:876–883.

SECTION 6

The Gastrointestinal Tract

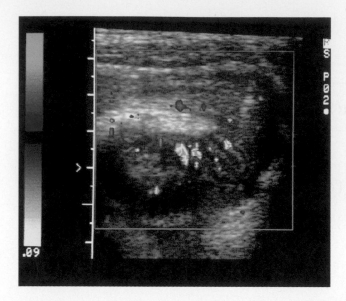

FIG. 96A. Patient 1.

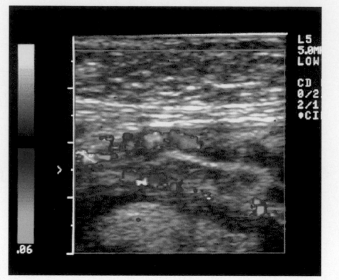

FIG. 96B. Patient 2.

History

Two different patients, aged 24 and 36, both with right lower-quadrant pain and possible appendicitis.

Findings

Figures 96A and B are transverse color Doppler sonograms of the right lower quadrant. Note the marked mural thickening of the terminal ileum and increased vascular flow within the wall of the terminal ileum in both patients.

Diagnosis

Crohn's disease of the terminal ileum in two patients.

Discussion

A thickened segment of bowel identified on grayscale imaging is a very nonspecific finding that may be caused by inflammation, ischemia, intramural hemorrhage, or tumor. The demonstration of increased flow within this focal segment strongly suggests inflammation or infection, and strongly argues against ischemia or infarction as the most likely diagnosis. It is not uncommon for patients with Crohn's disease to show signs and symptoms of appendicitis initially, as in the two patients in this case. Surgery is generally contraindicated in acute Crohn's disease because most patients can be successfully managed medically. It is important, however, to conduct careful air-contrast barium studies to document the extent of involvement of the gastrointestinal tract with Crohn's disease. The differential diagnosis includes other forms of infectious ileitis such as *Campylobacter*, *Salmonella*, tuberculosis, and *Yersinia* enteritis. The color Doppler findings are nonspecific for Crohn's and can be abnormal in all of these entities.

References

Jeffrey RB Jr, Sommer FG, Debatin JF. Color Doppler sonography of focal gastrointestinal lesions: initial clinical experience. *J Ultrasound Med* 1994;13:473–478.

Matsumoto T, Iida M, Sakai T, Kimura Y, Fujishima M. *Yersinia* terminal ileitis: sonographic findings in eight patients. *AJR* 1991;156:965–967.

Quillin SP, Siegel MJ. Gastrointestinal inflammation in children: color Doppler ultrasonography. *J Ultrasound Med* 1994;13:751–756.

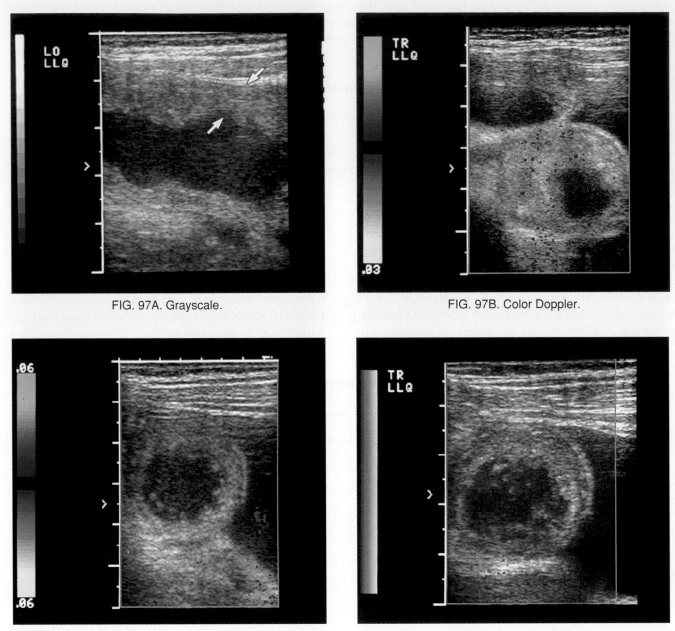

FIG. 97A. Grayscale.

FIG. 97B. Color Doppler.

FIG. 97C. Color Doppler.

FIG. 97D. Power Doppler.

History

Severe left lower-quadrant pain and questionable palpable mass.

Findings

Figure 97A, a longitudinal scan of the left lower quadrant, demonstrates marked mural thickening of a segment of small bowel (arrows). Figures 97B and C are transverse scans of the left lower quadrant with color Doppler imaging. Note that flow is absent in the thickened small bowel segments and surrounding ascites. Figure 97D, a power Doppler sonogram in a similar anatomic plane, demonstrates no intramural flow within the thickened segment of bowel.

Diagnosis

Closed-loop obstruction with bowel infarction.

Discussion

CT is the imaging method of choice in cases of possible small bowel obstruction and inconclusive plain radiographs. Because the patient had a palpable mass on physical examination, ultrasound was initially ordered. The "palpable mass" represented a focally thickened segment of bowel. With grayscale imaging, the differential diagnosis of focal bowel wall thickening is quite large and includes inflammation, ischemia, hemorrhage, and tumor. The absence of flow within the thickened bowel segment strongly favors the diagnosis of ischemia or infarction. At surgery, a closed-loop obstruction and infarction of the small bowel were found secondary to adhesions.

References

Jeffrey RB Jr, Sommer FG, Debatin JF. Color Doppler sonography of focal gastrointestinal lesions: initial clinical experience. *J Ultrasound Med* 1994;13:473–478.

Ko YT, Lim JH, Lee DH, Lee HW, Lim JW. Small bowel obstruction: sonographic evaluation. *Radiology* 1993;188:649–653.

Ogata M, Imai S, Hosotani R, Aoyama H, Hayashi M, Ishikawa T. Abdominal sonography for the diagnosis of large bowel obstruction. *Surg Today* 1994;24:791–794.

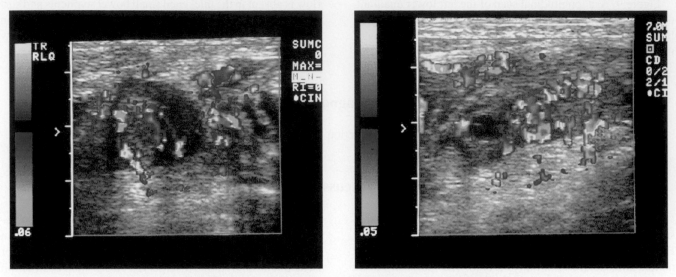

FIG. 98A. Color Doppler.

FIG. 98B. Color Doppler.

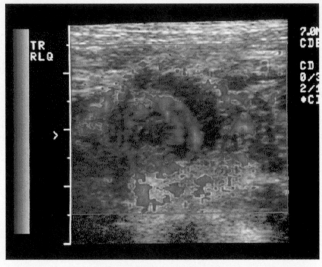

FIG. 98C. Power Doppler.

History

Right lower-quadrant pain for 10 days. Rule out pelvic inflammatory disease.

Findings

Figures 98A and B are transverse and longitudinal scans of the right lower quadrant that demonstrate marked mural thickening of the appendix with extensive hyperemia. Figure 98C is a power Doppler sonogram that confirms these findings and also demonstrates marked increased flow to the abnormally thickened appendix.

Diagnosis

Gangrenous appendicitis with marked hyperemia.

Discussion

The sonographic diagnosis of appendicitis is generally based on the grayscale findings of a noncompressible appendix that is >7 mm. Focal pain will often be elicited when the transducer is pressed directly over the appendix. Color Doppler sonography has a relatively minor role to play in the evaluation of these patients. In this patient, the finding of marked hyperemia of the appendiceal wall was communicated to the surgeon, who elected to perform an open appendectomy rather than attempt an appendectomy using a laparoscopic approach. Because of the difficult exposure via the laparoscopic method, open appendectomy may also be preferred in patients with perforated appendix. This case nicely illustrates that, with current high-resolution equipment, even small branches of the appendiceal artery can be clearly identified with color Doppler imaging. Avascular areas are likely to represent areas of infarction or abscess formation.

References

Quillin SP, Siegel MJ. Appendicitis: efficacy of color Doppler sonography. *Radiology* 1994;191:557–560.
Quillin SP, Siegel MJ. Diagnosis of appendiceal abscess in children with acute appendicitis: value of color Doppler sonography. *AJR* 1995;164:1251–1254.

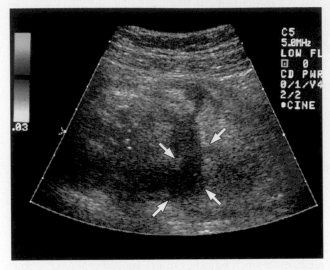

FIG. 99A. Color Doppler.

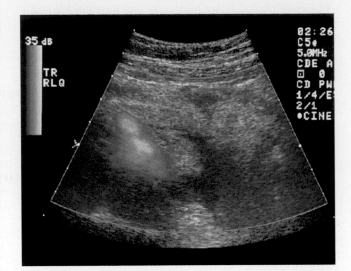

FIG. 99B. Power Doppler.

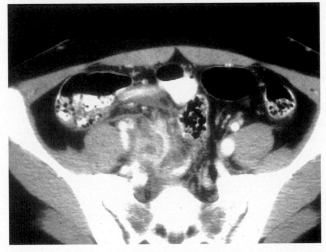

FIG. 99C. Contrast-enhanced CT.

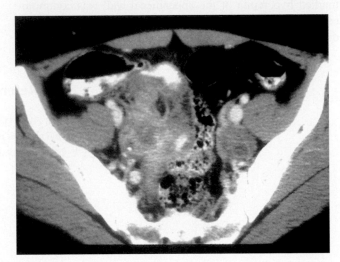

FIG. 99D. Contrast-enhanced CT.

History

Right lower-quadrant pain for 5 days. Rule out appendicitis.

Findings

Figure 99A, a color Doppler sonogram of the right lower quadrant, shows a hypoechoic area (arrows) surrounded by fat with increased echogenicity. There is relatively little flow with color Doppler imaging. Figure 99B is a power Doppler sonogram demonstrating marked hyperemia of the echogenic fat. Figures 99C and D are contrast-enhanced CT scans demonstrating a large mesenteric phlegmon with low-attenuation abscess formation centrally.

Diagnosis

Perforated appendicitis with mesenteric abscess and phlegmon.

Discussion

Power Doppler sonography in this patient clearly identified the mesenteric hyperemia associated with perforated appendicitis. Because these vessels are often 1 to 2 mm in size, they are not readily imaged with conventional color Doppler. The avascular areas represent liquefied pus and abscess formation surrounded by the echogenic inflamed mesenteric fat. These findings were confirmed on contrast-enhanced CT.

The inflamed mesenteric phlegmon is enhanced significantly more than adjacent muscle. Because of the relatively small abscess and the large surrounding phlegmon, this patient was treated conservatively with antibiotics and discharged 5 days later on oral antibiotics. An interval appendectomy was performed electively 6 weeks later through a clean operative field following the resolution of the mesenteric phlegmon.

References

Quillin SP, Siegel MJ. Appendicitis: efficacy of color Doppler sonography. *Radiology* 1994,191.557 560
Quillin SP, Siegel MJ. Diagnosis of appendiceal abscess in children with acute appendicitis: value of color Doppler sonography. *AJR* 1995;164:1251–1254.

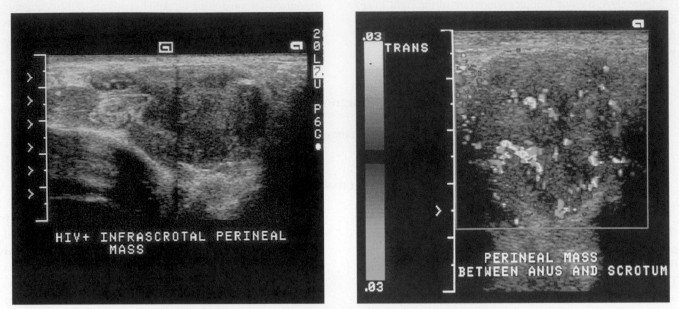

FIG. 100A. Grayscale.

FIG. 100B. Color Doppler.

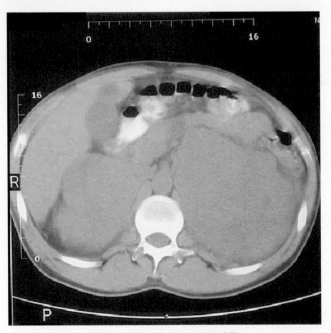

FIG. 100C. Noncontrast CT.

History

A 34-year-old HIV-positive male with a tender and painful perineal mass between the anus and scrotum, and with a CD4 lymphocyte count of 23.

Findings

Figure 100A, a longitudinal compound image of the infrascrotal perineal mass, reveals a mixed-echogenicity, predominantly hypoechoic mass that measures 6.5 × 4.0 × 4.0 cm. Figure 100B, a transverse color Doppler sonogram of the mass, reveals prominent internal flow throughout the mass.

Ultrasound-guided biopsy revealed lymphoma, later classified on immunohistochemistry analysis as a high-grade B-cell lymphoma. Figure 100C, a noncontrast CT scan at the level of the kidneys, reveals marked bilateral renal involvement by the lymphoma.

Diagnosis

HIV-related lymphoma.

Discussion

An HIV-positive patient with a CD4 count of <200 is, by the current Centers for Disease Control definition, a patient with AIDS. Several types of lymphoma have a much higher prevalence in HIV-positive patients than in the general population. Primary gastric and primary CNS lymphoma are much more common in HIV-positive patients. Moderate- to high-grade B-cell lymphomas are AIDS-defining conditions. Hodgkin's lymphoma and other non-Hodgkin's lymphomas are not AIDS-defining conditions and have no higher prevalence in HIV-positive patients than in the general population. Of course, because of the severe immunologic compromise in HIV-positive patients, these lymphomas often involve much more aggressive and advanced disease. All HIV-related lymphomas should be considered disseminated when diagnosed, even if only one site is identified clinically or by imaging. Unusual presentations, such as this perineal mass, are not infrequent. The staging noncontrast CT (the patient was discovered to have mild renal failure) revealed bilateral renal involvement. Some low-attenuation areas in the tip of the right lobe of the liver suggested the possibility of hepatic involvement, as well. This patient also had extensive retroperitoneal and pelvic adenopathy.

Reference

Radin DR, Esplin JA, Levine AM, et al. AIDS related non-Hodgkin's lymphoma: abdominal CT findings in 112 patients. *AJR* 1993;160:1133.

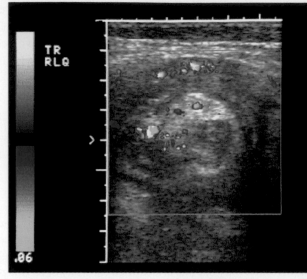

FIG. 101A. Color Doppler.

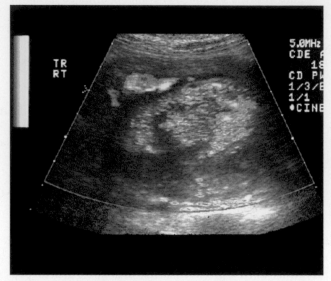

FIG. 101B. Power Doppler.

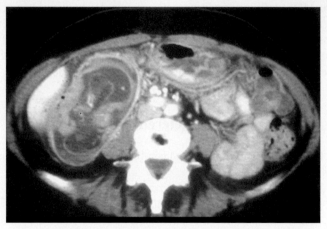

FIG. 101C. Contrast-enhanced CT.

History

Right lower-quadrant pain with palpable mass. Rule out periappendiceal abscess.

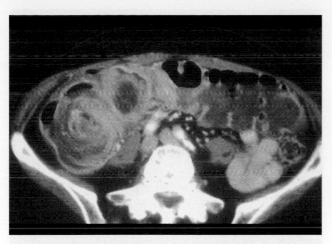

FIG. 101D. Contrast-enhanced CT..

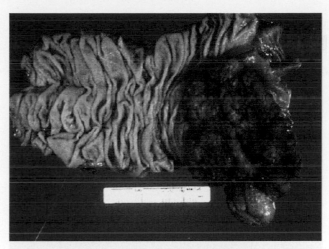

FIG. 101E. Pathology specimen.

Findings

Figure 101A is a transverse color Doppler sonogram showing a complex mass in the right lower quadrant. Note that the inner component appears echogenic and the outer component appears hypoechoic. Figure 101B is a power Doppler sonogram revealing that the inner echogenic component is quite vascular. Figures 101C and D are contrast-enhanced CT scans demonstrating a colocolonic intussusception. Figure 101E is the resected gross pathology specimen showing a cecal carcinoma as the lead point.

Diagnosis

Colocolonic intussusception from cecal carcinoma.

Discussion

In this patient, grayscale imaging revealed a nonspecific complex right lower-quadrant mass. The inner echogenic component of this mass represented invaginated mesenteric fat. The vessels adjacent to the fat (identified on both color and power Doppler sonography) were the invaginated ileocolic vessels of the right colon. Although the lead point (in this case, a cecal carcinoma) was not identified, an intussusception was suspected based on the sonographic findings. The color Doppler appearance of the mesenteric vessels of the intussusceptum and the mural vascularity of the intussusceptions were helpful to establish the diagnosis.

References

Lam AH, Firman K. Value of sonography including color Doppler in the diagnosis and management of long standing intussusception. *Pediatr Radiol* 1992;22:112–114.

Lim JH, Ko YT, Lee HW, Lim JW. Determining the site and causes of colonic obstruction with sonography. *AJR* 1994;165:1113–1117.

Weinberger E, Winters WD. Intussusception in children: the role of sonography. *Radiology* 1992;184:601–602.

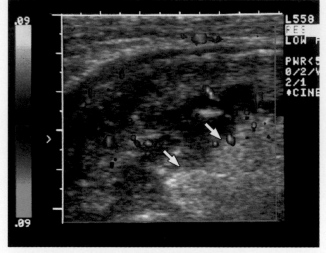

FIG. 102A. Color Doppler.

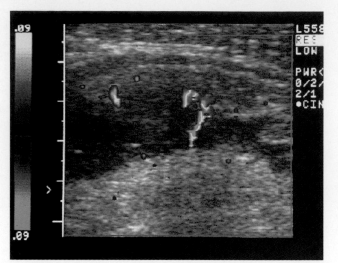

FIG. 102B. Color Doppler.

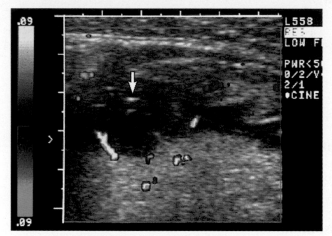

FIG. 102C. Color Doppler.

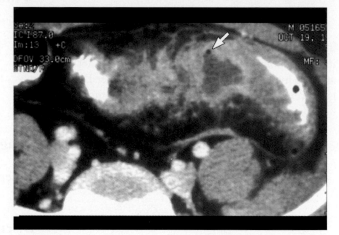

FIG. 102D. Contrast-enhanced CT.

History

A 64-year-old male with left lower-quadrant pain and fever. Rule out abscess.

Findings

Figures 102A–C are transverse scans of the left lower quadrant that demonstrate marked mural thickening of the descending colon. Note the prominent echogenic fat adjacent to the thickened bowel (arrows). Areas of hyperemia are noted with increased vascular flow. In Fig. 102C, a focal area of linear high-amplitude echogenicity corresponds to a gas bubble within the thickened colonic wall (arrow). Figure 102D is a contrast-enhanced CT demonstrating marked mural thickening of the descending colon with a well-defined low-attenuation abscess containing a gas bubble (arrow).

Diagnosis

Acute diverticulitis with paracolonic abscess formation.

Discussion

CT and contrast enemas are generally the imaging methods of choice to evaluate patients with left lower-quadrant pain and suspected diverticulitis. On occasion, however, sonography may be performed in patients who have atypical signs and symptoms. The sonographic hallmarks include mural thickening of the sigmoid colon (noncompressible with the graded-compression technique), increased echogenicity in the paracolonic fat due to edema and inflammation, hypoechoic paracolonic abscesses, and increased mural vascularity cause by hyperemia and inflammation.

References

Nuako KW, Gostout NJ. Sonography in acute colonic diverticulitis. *Am J Gastroenterol* 1994;89:455–456.
Schwerk WB, Schwarz S, Rothmund M. Sonography in acute colonic diverticulitis: a prospective study. *Dis Colon Rectum* 1992;35:1077–1084.
Yacoe ME, Jeffrey RB Jr. Sonography of appendicitis and diverticulitis. *Radiol Clin North Am* 1994;32:899–912.

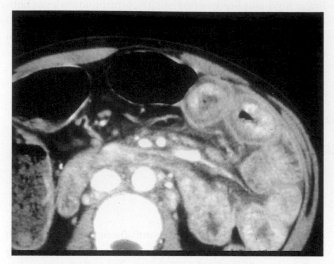

FIG. 103A. Contrast-enhanced CT.

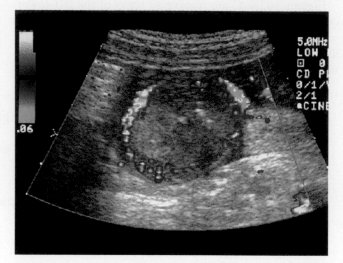

FIG. 103B. Color Doppler.

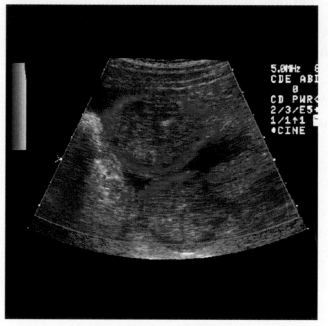

FIG. 103C. Power Doppler.

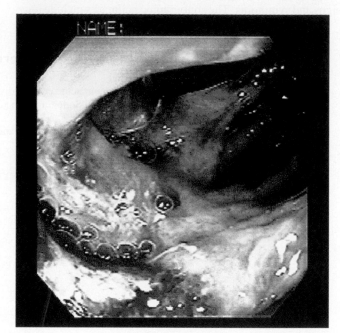

FIG. 103D. Small bowel endoscopy.

History

A 39-year-old female with systemic lupus erythematosus and acute left upper-quadrant pain.

Findings

Figure 103A is a contrast-enhanced CT showing mural thickening of multiple loops of proximal jejunum in the left upper quadrant. Figures 103B and C, color and power Doppler sonograms of these bowel loops, demonstrate excellent flow to the bowel wall. Figure 103D is small bowel endoscopy demonstrating purplish areas of petechial hemorrhage of the mucosal surface, but no evidence of transmural infarction.

Diagnosis

Jejunal vasculitis secondary to lupus erythematosus.

Discussion

In this patient with acute abdominal pain, the CT findings of thickened bowel wall and submucosal edema were nonspecific and could have represented infarction or ischemia. However, the ability to demonstrate perfusion to the bowel wall with color and power Doppler was helpful in suggesting that there was only small vessel involvement and not transmural infarction of the bowel. This was confirmed with small bowel endoscopy that demonstrated patchy areas of mucosal ischemia, but no evidence of infarction. Biopsy revealed early changes of vasculitis. The color Doppler and power Doppler findings in this case clearly affected patient management and prevented early laparotomy. The patient was treated with a bolus of steroids and rapidly recovered.

References

Jeffrey RB Jr, Sommer FG, Debatin JF. Color Doppler sonography of focal gastrointestinal lesions: initial clinical experience. *J Ultrasound Med* 1994;13:473–478.

Matsumoto T, Iida M, Sakai T, Kimura Y, Fujishima M. *Yersinia* terminal ileitis: sonographic findings in eight patients. *AJR* 1991;156:965–967.

Quillin SP, Siegel MJ. Gastrointestinal inflammation in children: color Doppler ultrasonography. *J Ultrasound Med* 1994;13:751–756.

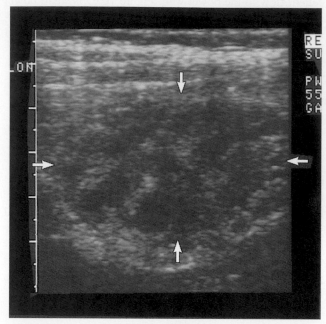

FIG. 104A. Grayscale.

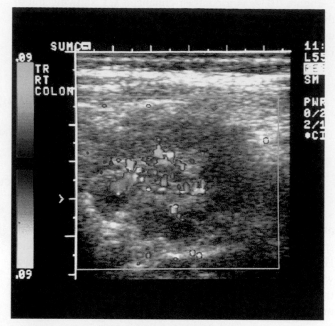

FIG. 104B. Color Doppler.

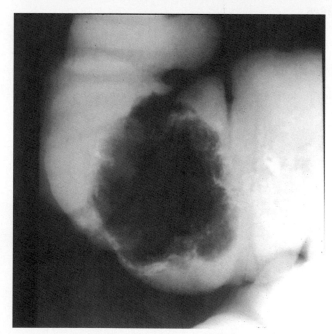

FIG. 104C. Barium enema.

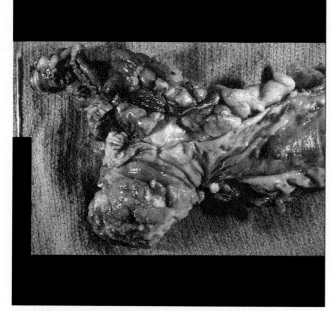

FIG. 104D. Pathology specimen.

History

A 70-year-old male with vague right lower-quadrant pain. Rule out appendicitis.

Findings

Figure 104A, a grayscale sonogram of the right lower quadrant, reveals an ill-defined hypoechoic mass (arrows). Figure 104B is a color Doppler sonogram demonstrating internal flow within the hypoechoic mass radiating out in a spoke-wheel fashion. Figure 104C is a single-contrast barium enema showing a large polypoid lesion in the right colon. Figure 104D is a pathologic specimen demonstrating the large villous adenoma of the cecum.

Diagnosis

Villous adenoma of the cecum presenting as right lower-quadrant pain.

Discussion

In patients >40 years of age, neoplasm must always be considered in the differential diagnosis of right lower-quadrant pain and possible appendicitis. In this patient, a nonspecific hypoechoic mass was identified with grayscale imaging. Intrinsic color Doppler flow within the mass suggested a solid lesion and not an abscess. Although a specific diagnosis could not be established on the basis of the ultrasound alone, neoplasm was strongly considered. This was confirmed by a barium enema study and subsequently at surgery. Other neoplasms that may present in the right lower quadrant include cecal carcinoma, lymphoma, cecal implants from metastatic disease, and Ewing's sarcoma of the iliac fossa. This patient's pain may have been caused by intermittent intussusception.

References

Jeffrey RB Jr, Sommer FG, Debatin JF. Color Doppler sonography of focal gastrointestinal lesions: initial clinical experience. *J Ultrasound Med* 1994;13:473–478.

Matsumoto T, Iida M, Sakai T, Kimura Y, Fujishima M. *Yersinia* terminal ileitis: sonographic findings in eight patients. *AJR* 1991;156:965–967.

Quillin SP, Siegel MJ. Gastrointestinal inflammation in children: color Doppler ultrasonography. *J Ultrasound Med* 1994;13:751–756.

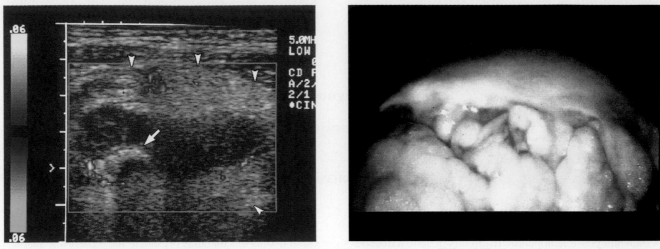

FIG. 105A. Color Doppler.

FIG. 105B. Laparoscopy.

History

A 23-year-old male who had 5 days of right lower-quadrant pain and fever. Rule out appendicitis.

Findings

Figure 105A, a transverse scan of the right lower quadrant, demonstrates a large noncompressible appendix containing an appendicolith (arrow) at its base. Notice the prominent echogenic fat (arrowheads) surrounding the appendix that contains vascularized flow on color Doppler. Figure 105B is a still frame taken from laparoscopy demonstrating the inflamed omentum extending over the right lower quadrant.

Diagnosis

Gangrenous appendicitis with adherent omentum.

Discussion

Inflamed intra-abdominal fat is often echogenic and demonstrates intrinsic vascularity with low-volume flow sensitivity on color Doppler sonography. This may be true of the inflamed omentum around the gallbladder in patients with acute cholecystitis or the inflamed mesentery and omentum in cases of gangrenous appendicitis. The loss of the echogenic submucosal layer of the appendiceal wall and the prominent surrounding echogenic fat are consistent with gangrenous appendicitis. The laparoscopic resection was quite difficult and lengthy because of the adherent omentum. Because of the difficulty of laparoscopic dissection, this case may have better been treated by open laparotomy. Recognition of inflamed omentum encasing the right lower quadrant, therefore, may be important preoperative information in guiding the decision planning of open versus laparoscopic appendectomy.

References

Jeffrey RB Jr, Sommer FG, Debatin JF. Color Doppler sonography of focal gastrointestinal lesions: initial clinical experience. *J Ultrasound Med* 1994;13:473–478.

Matsumoto T, Iida M, Sakai T, Kimura Y, Fujishima M. *Yersinia* terminal ileitis: sonographic findings in eight patients. *AJR* 1991;156:965–967.

Quillin SP, Siegel MJ. Gastrointestinal inflammation in children: color Doppler ultrasonography. *J Ultrasound Med* 1994;13:751–756.

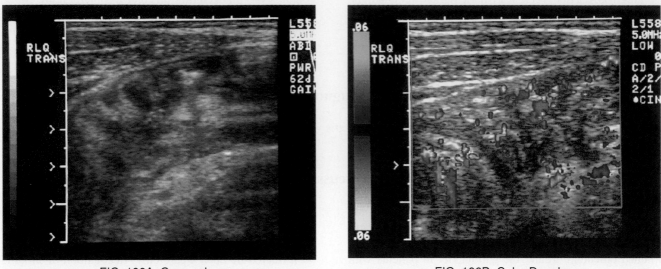

FIG. 106A. Grayscale.

FIG. 106B. Color Doppler.

History

A 23-year-old female with right lower-quadrant pain and diarrhea 2 weeks after oral antibiotic therapy for tonsillitis.

Findings

Figure 106A, a transverse scan of the right lower quadrant, demonstrates a noncompressible and thickened ascending colon. Figure 106B is a color Doppler sonogram demonstrating increased flow within the right colon.

Diagnosis

Pseudomembranous colitis.

Discussion

The identification of thickening of the right colon with increased flow with color Doppler was the key to the diagnosis. The history of prior antibiotic therapy led to a presumptive diagnosis of pseudomembranous colitis, which was confirmed with stool cultures. Not all patients with pseudomembranous colitis develop diarrhea, and some patients present predominantly with fever and abdominal pain mimicking an abscess. Identification of thickened segments of colon was therefore very important in suggesting the diagnosis. This is further underscored by the demonstration of increased flow with color Doppler sonography.

References

Boland GW, Lee MJ, Cats AM, Ferraro MJ, Matthia AR, Mueller PR. *Clostridium difficile* colitis: correlation of CT findings with severity of clinical disease. *Clin Radiol* 1995;50:153–156.

Boland GW, Lee MJ, Cats AM, Gaa JA, Saini S, Mueller PR. Antibiotic-induced diarrhea: specificity of abdominal CT for the diagnosis of *Clostridium difficile* disease. *Radiology* 1994;191:103–106.

Jacobs JE, Birnbaum BA. CT of inflammatory disease of the colon. *Semin Ultrasound CT MR* 1995;16:91–101.

Section 7

The Female Pelvis

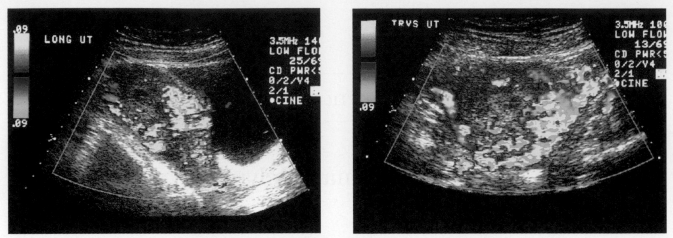

FIG. 107A. Color Doppler.　　　　　　　　FIG. 107B. Color Doppler.

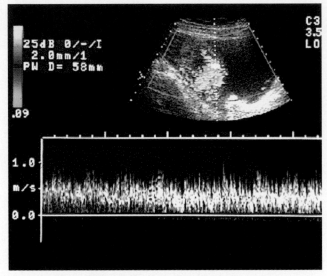

FIG. 107C. Doppler spectrum.

History

A 42-year-old female who, after multiple prior dilatation and curettage procedures, was infertile and had repeated first-pregnancy miscarriages.

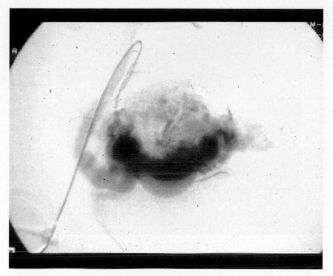

FIG. 107D. Arteriogram.

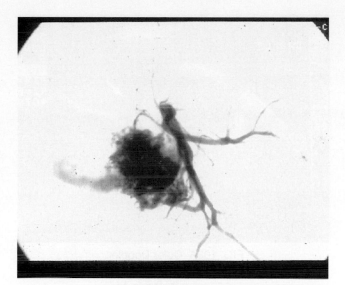

FIG. 107E. Arteriogram.

Findings

Figures 107A and B are longitudinal and transverse color Doppler sonograms of the uterus that demonstrate marked hypervascularity of the corpus of the uterus and adnexa (Fig. 107D). Figure 107C is a spectral Doppler tracing that demonstrates pulsatile venous flow. Figures 107D and E are selective internal iliac arteriograms demonstrating a uterine arteriovenous fistula.

Diagnosis

Uterine arteriovenous fistula

Discussion

Arteriovenous fistulas of the uterus and vagina are quite rare, but may be caused by prior surgical procedures such as prior dilatation and curettage, as in this case. Other etiologies include congenital fistulas or fistulas caused by tumor invasion of uterine arteries. Color Doppler sonography plays a pivotal role in the diagnosis of these fistulas by demonstrating a vascular mass containing pulsatile venous flow. Undoubtedly the arteriovenous fistula caused a "steal phenomenon" from the endometrial cavity, resulting in endometrial ischemia and repeated early-pregnancy miscarriages. Treatment options include both selective catheter embolization and/or surgery following embolization. The identification of the uterine arteriovenous fistula in this patient was of critical importance, because further instrumentation may have resulted in exsanguinating hemorrhage.

Reference

Jain KA, Jeffrey RB Jr, Sommer FG. Gynecologic vascular abnormalities: diagnosis with Doppler ultrasound. *Radiology* 1991;178:549–551.

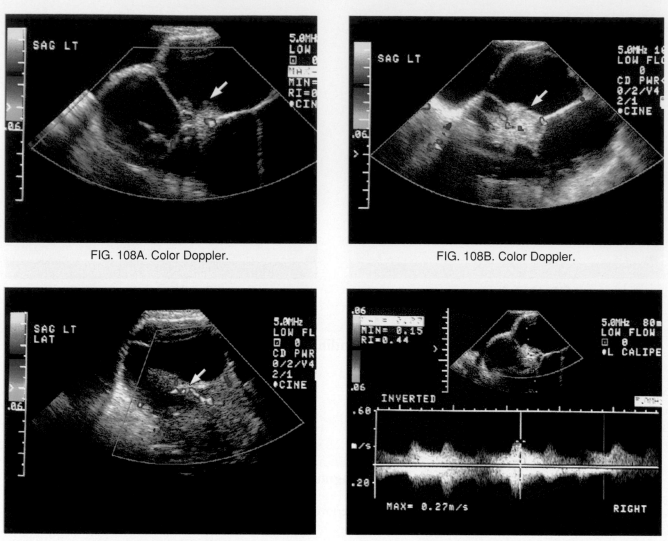

FIG. 108A. Color Doppler.

FIG. 108B. Color Doppler.

FIG. 108C. Color Doppler.

FIG. 108D. Doppler spectrum.

History

A 60-year-old female with pelvic fullness. Rule out adnexal mass.

Findings

Figures 108A–D are endovaginal color Doppler sonograms. Note that, in Figs. 108A–C, there is a complex cystic mass containing multiple septations (arrows), and a vascularized septal nodule is seen centrally. A spectral Doppler tracing from this mass demonstrates a resistive index (RI) of 0.44.

Diagnosis

Ovarian carcinoma.

Discussion

One of the main values of color Doppler sonography in the evaluation of pelvic masses is the identification of vascularized septal nodules. This finding is highly suggestive of a malignant ovarian neoplasm. Many benign complex cysts will have "solid" components within them that are areas of hemorrhage, clot, debris, etc., that will be avascular with color Doppler sonography. Some authors have suggested that an RI < 0.40 strongly correlates with malignant neoplasm. The RI in this case was borderline at 0.44. Thus, a single numerical value is of only marginal help in the management of these patients. The most important features in determining benign from malignant ovarian masses are size (>6 cm strongly correlates with neoplasm) and morphology. The morphologic features suggesting malignancy include septal or mural nodules that have vascular flow detectable with color Doppler sonography.

References

Brown DL, Frates MC, Laing FC, et al. Ovarian masses: can benign and malignant lesions be differentiated with color and pulsed Doppler US? *Radiology* 1994;190:333–336.

Carter J, Saltzman A, Hartenbach E, Fowler J, Carson L, Twiggs LB. Flow characteristics in benign and malignant gynecologic tumors using transvaginal color flow Doppler. *Obstet Gynecol* 1994;83:125–130.

Kurjak A, Predanic M, Kupesic-Urek S, Jukic S. Transvaginal color and pulsed Doppler assessment of adnexal tumor vascularity. *Gynecol Oncol* 1993;50:3–9.

Stein SM, Laifer-Narin S, Johnson MB, et al. Differentiation of benign and malignant adnexal masses: relative value of gray-scale, color Doppler, and spectral Doppler sonography. *AJR* 1995;164:381–386.

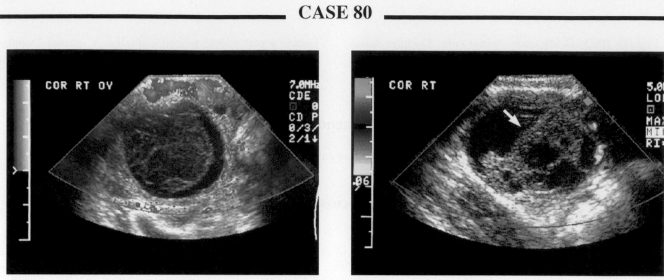

FIG. 109A. Patient 1.

FIG. 109B. Patient 2.

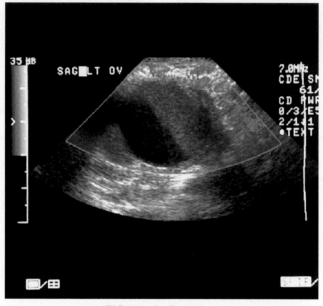

FIG. 109C. Patient 3.

History

Three different patients with similar etiologies of an adnexal mass.

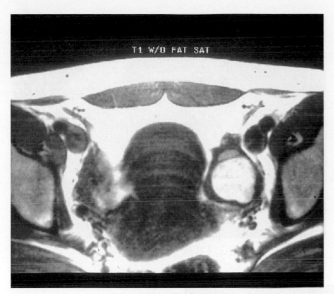

FIG. 109D. Patient 3.

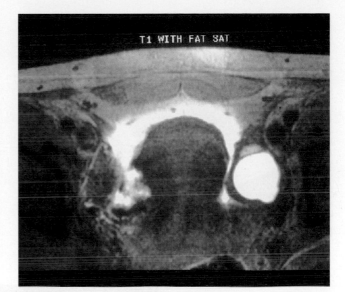

FIG. 109E. Patient 3.

Findings

Figures 109A–C are scans from three different patients with pelvic masses discovered on routine physical examination. Figure 109A demonstrates a "fishnet" pattern of fine interdigitating strands. Note that, with power Doppler sonography, there is no internal flow within the mass. Figure 109B is another patient with an adnexal mass also demonstrating no flow internally within the mass. Note the straight edge (ar-row) of debris within the mass. Figure 109C is an endovaginal power Doppler sonogram demonstrating a fluid–fluid level that is also avascular. This same patient underwent an MRI study (Figs. 109D and E). Note the high-signal left adnexal mass that remains high signal on T1-weighted images without (Fig. 109D) and with (Fig. 109E) fat suppression.

Diagnosis

Hemorrhagic ovarian cysts in three patients.

Discussion

Hemorrhagic ovarian cysts are common in clinical practice. The importance in identifying macroscopic hemorrhage within a cyst is that it is rarely caused by carcinoma and generally indicates a benign lesion that can be followed clinically or with sonography. Ovarian carcinomas can, very rarely, however, rupture and cause hemoperitoneum. Hemorrhage in patients receiving anticoagulant therapy may rarely cause an ovarian cyst. Hemorrhage most often occurs in functional cysts and endometriomas. A variety of sonographic patterns may be seen with hemorrhagic cysts. However, hemorrhage will invariably be avascular with color Doppler and power Doppler. Figure 109A demonstrates a "fishnet" pattern of interlacing strands of fibrin. Figure 109B demonstrates evidence of avascular clot within the cystic mass. In Fig. 109C is a fluid–fluid level representing a hematocrit effect. MRI may be very useful in selected cases to confirm hemorrhage within an adnexal mass. High signal within the mass will be evident on T1-weighted images with and without fat saturation.

References

Geisler JP, Denman BJ, Cudahy TJ, Lee TH, Geisler HE. Ovarian carcinoma presenting as intra-abdominal hemorrhage. *Gynecol Oncol* 1994;53:380–381.

Outwater E, Schiebler ML, Owen RS, Schnall MD. Characterization of hemorrhagic adnexal lesions with MR imaging: blinded reader study. *Radiology* 1993;186:489–494.

Wilbur AC, Goldstein LD, Prywitch BA. Hemorrhagic ovarian cysts in patients on anticoagulation therapy: CT findings. *J Comput Assist Tomogr* 1993;17:623–625.

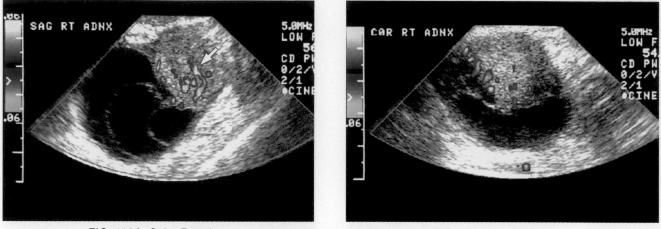

FIG. 110A. Color Doppler.

FIG. 110B. Color Doppler.

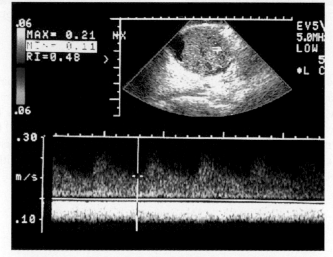

FIG. 110C. Doppler spectrum.

History

A 49-year-old female with a right adnexal mass on physical examination.

Findings

Figures 110A–C are color Doppler endovaginal sonograms. In Figs. 110A and B is a complex cystic mass that demonstrates solid components. Note the intrinsic vascularity within the solid mural nodule (arrow, Fig. 110A). Thin septae are seen within the more cystic component of the mass. Figure 110C is a spectral Doppler tracing that demonstrates a low resistive index.

Diagnosis

Ovarian carcinoma.

Discussion

This case illustrates a characteristic feature of ovarian carcinoma: vascularized mural nodules. This finding alone has such high specificity for a neoplasm that it indicates the need for surgery. Benign neoplasms, such as cystic teratomas (dermoids), may rarely contain solid vascularized tissue in the wall of the cystic mass (i.e., ectopic thyroid tissue). The attempt to characterize adnexal masses solely on the basis of Doppler waveform analysis has met with mixed results. Malignant masses typically have central flow within a solid portion of the mass (septal or mural nodule) and low impedance. Benign ovarian masses typically demonstrate peripheral flow with high impedance. Unfortunately, there is often significant overlap between these two Doppler categories. Most authorities now agree that morphologic and Doppler features must be analyzed in combination to achieve the most accurate results in distinguishing benign from malignant ovarian masses.

References

Fleischer AC, Rodgers WH, Kepple DM, Williams LL, Jones HW III. Color Doppler sonography of ovarian masses: a multiparameter analysis. *J Ultrasound Med* 1993;12:41–48.

Kurjak A, Zalud I, Alfirevic Z. Evaluation of adnexal masses with transvaginal color ultrasound. *J Ultrasound Med* 1991;10:295–297.

Salem S, White LM, Lai J. Doppler sonography of adnexal masses: the predictive value of the pulsatility index in benign and malignant disease. *AJR* 1994;163:1147–1150.

Stein SM, Laifer-Narin S, Johnson MB, et al. Differentiation of benign and malignant adnexal masses: relative value of gray-scale, color Doppler, and spectral Doppler sonography. *AJR* 1995;164:381–386.

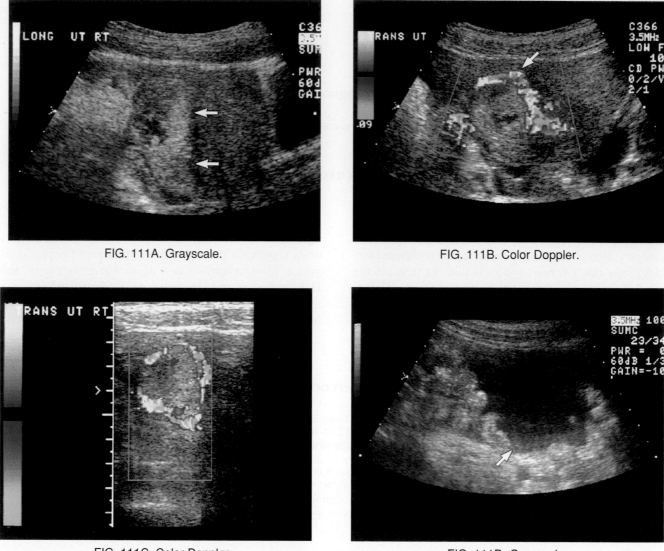

FIG. 111A. Grayscale.

FIG. 111B. Color Doppler.

FIG. 111C. Color Doppler.

FIG. 111D. Grayscale.

History

A 27-year-old female with right lower-quadrant pain and positive β human chorionic gonadotropin. Rule out ectopic pregnancy.

Findings

Figure 111A, a grayscale sonogram of the uterus, demonstrates no evidence of an intrauterine pregnancy. Echogenic fluid (hemoperitoneum) is seen posterior to the uterus (arrows). Figure 111B, a transverse scan of the uterus, shows an echogenic mass involving the right lateral contour of the uterus. Notice that, with color Doppler, there is prominent increased flow around the periphery of the mass (arrow). This finding is again demonstrated in Fig. 111C, as increased color Doppler flow is seen on the periphery of this echogenic mass. Figure 111D, a sagittal scan of the left lower quadrant, demonstrates a large amount of complex intraperitoneal fluid (arrow).

Diagnosis

Ruptured interstitial (cornual) ectopic pregnancy.

Discussion

Interstitial or cornual ectopic pregnancies are relatively rare and represent only 2% to 3% of all ectopic pregnancies. Unlike tubal pregnancies that typically rupture at 6 to 8 weeks of gestational age, it is not uncommon for interstitial pregnancies to rupture much later in pregnancy, because there is abundant blood supply from the myometrium to support the pregnancy and perhaps greater distensibility of the myometrium than the tube to accommodate the enlarging gestational sac. Thus, the mortality in a ruptured interstitial pregnancy in some reports has been noted to be twice that for patients with tubal ectopic pregnancies. The sonographic hallmark of an interstitial pregnancy is a gestational sac or echogenic mass localized eccentrically along the margin of the uterus. In some patients, a thin echogenic line (the interstitial line) may be noted connecting the myometrial cavity to the interstitial ectopic. There may be thinning of the myometrium, as in this case. As with other forms of ectopic pregnancy, color Doppler sonography may demonstrate prominent increased peritrophoblastic flow, euphemistically referred to as the "ring of fire." Spectral Doppler tracings will demonstrate high diastolic flow in these regions because of low-impedance flow.

References

Ackerman TE, Levi CS, Dashefsky SM, Holt SC, Linday DJ. Interstitial line: sonographic finding in interstitial (cornual) ectopic pregnancy. *Radiology* 1993;189:83–87.

Ackerman TE, Levi CS, Lyons EA. US case of the day: right-sided interstitial (cornual) ectopic pregnancy. *Radiographics* 1994;14:185–187.

Chen GD, Lin MT, Lee MS. Diagnosis of interstitial pregnancy with sonography. *J Clin Ultrasound* 1994; 22:439–442.

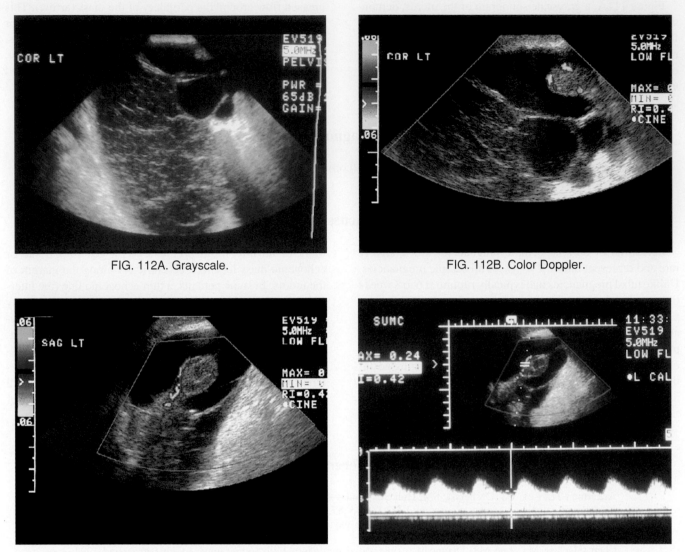

FIG. 112A. Grayscale.

FIG. 112B. Color Doppler.

FIG. 112C. Color Doppler.

FIG. 112D. Doppler spectrum.

History

A 72-year-old female with a large pelvic mass on pelvic examination.

Findings

Figure 112A, a coronal endovaginal scan of a left adnexal mass, demonstrates multiple thin septations. Figures 112B and C are color Doppler endovaginal sonograms demonstrating vascularized septal nodules. Figure 112D is a spectral Doppler tracing obtained from a vessel traversing a septation demonstrating a resistive index of 0.42.

Diagnosis

Ovarian carcinoma with vascularized septal nodules.

Discussion

The low-level echoes and thin septations seen in Fig. 112A mimic the "fishnet" pattern of interlacing strands of fibrin typical of hemorrhagic cysts. However, hemorrhagic cysts are avascular and do not demonstrate flow within septal nodules, which are evident in this case. This finding alone strongly indicates an ovarian neoplasm. Note that the resistive index (0.42) was slightly greater than the published threshold for malignancy of 0.40. Thus, the overall usefulness of resistive indices in the evaluation of adnexal masses must be called into question because very specific morphologic features of malignancy often take precedence over any single quantitative analysis of the Doppler waveform.

References

Fleischer AC, Rodgers WH, Kepple DM, Williams LL, Jones HW III. Color Doppler sonography of ovarian masses: a multiparameter analysis. *J Ultrasound Med* 1993;12:41–48.

Kurjack A, Zalud I, Alfirevic Z. Evaluation of adnexal masses with transvaginal color ultrasound. *J Ultrasound Med* 1991;10:295–297.

Salem S, White LM, Lai J. Doppler sonography of adnexal masses: the predictive value of the pulsatility index in benign and malignant disease. *AJR* 1994;163:1147–1150.

Stein SM, Laifer-Narin S, Johnson MB, et al. Differentiation of benign and malignant adnexal masses: relative value of gray-scale, color Doppler, and spectral Doppler sonography. *AJR* 1995;164:381–386.

CASE 84

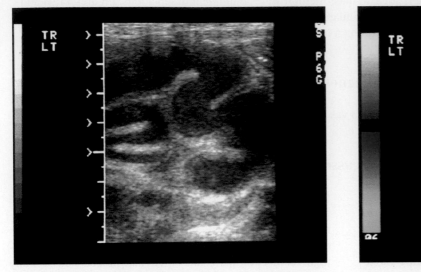

FIG. 113A. Grayscale.

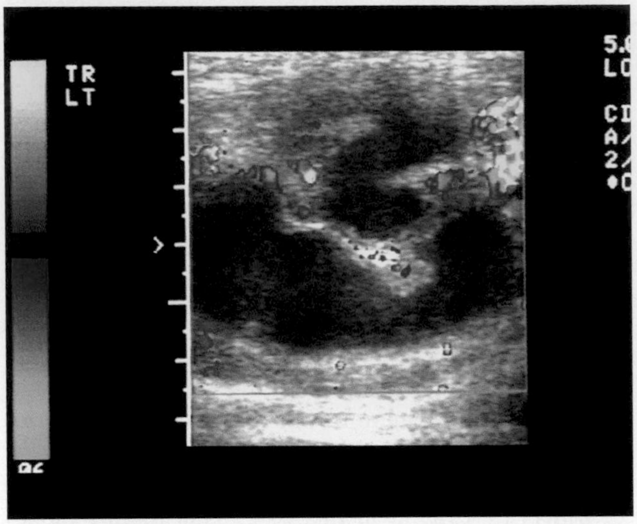

FIG. 113B. Color Doppler.

History

A 29-year-old female with left adnexal fullness.

Findings

Figure 113A, a grayscale image of the left adnexa, reveals a serpiginous hypoechoic mass. Figure 113B is a color Doppler sonogram demonstrating no vascular flow within the mass, indicating that it represents a hydrosalpinx.

Diagnosis

Left hydrosalpinx.

Discussion

With grayscale imaging alone, the serpiginous mass in the left adnexa could have been misdiagnosed as a vascular structure such as a pelvic varix. The fact that it contained no flow on color Doppler sonography strongly suggested the diagnosis of a hydrosalpinx. No further workup was required and, because of the patient's lack of symptoms, no further imaging studies were performed. Color Doppler sonography can be quite valuable in differentiating pelvic varices from a hydrosalpinx.

References

Atri M, Tran CN, Bret PM, Aidis AE, Kintzen GM. Accuracy of endovaginal sonography for the detection of fallopian tube blockage. *J Ultrasound Med* 1994;13:429–434.

Bulas DI, Ahlstrom PA, Sivit CJ, Blask AR, O'Donnell RM. Pelvic inflammatory disease in the adolescent: comparison of transabdominal and transvaginal sonographic evaluation. *Radiology* 1992;183:435–439.

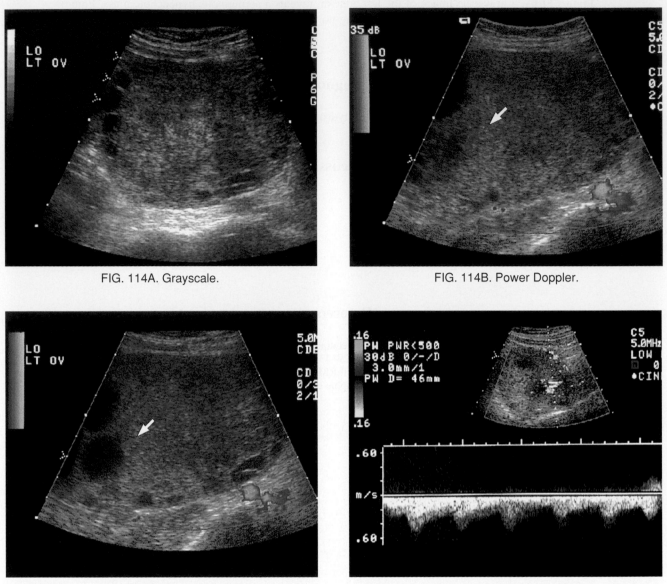

FIG. 114A. Grayscale.

FIG. 114B. Power Doppler.

FIG. 114C. Power Doppler.

FIG. 114D. Doppler spectrum.

History

A 24-year-old female with sudden onset of left lower-quadrant pain and palpable left adnexal mass. Rule out torsion.

Findings

Figure 114A, a grayscale sonogram of the left adnexa, shows an enlarged echogenic left ovary with prominent peripheral follicles. Figures 114B and C are power Doppler sonograms demonstrating some residual internal flow (arrows) within the enlarged left ovary. Figure 114D is a spectral Doppler tracing that reveals residual arterial flow within the enlarged ovary. No venous flow was evident.

Diagnosis

Ovarian torsion with preserved arterial flow.

Discussion

At surgery, this patient had a 360° torsed left ovary that was hemorrhagic and required surgical resection. Areas of infarction were noted pathologically. Because of the dual arterial blood supply to the ovaries (one branch from the aorta and another branch from the uterine arteries), it is very difficult to occlude arterial inflow to the ovary totally. Therefore, the identification of arterial vascularity does not exclude the diagnosis of ovarian torsion. The first vessels to be occluded are the low-pressure ovarian veins. The preservation of central venous flow has been noted by some authors to be a good sign for viability of the ovary. With grayscale imaging, the hallmark of torsion is ovarian enlargement with increased echogenicity caused by hemorrhage and congestion. Because of transudation of fluid, prominent peripheral follicles are also a characteristic feature of ovarian torsion.

References

Fleischer AC, Culinan JA, Kepple DM, Williams LL. Conventional and color Doppler transvaginal sonography of pelvic masses: a comparison of relative histologic specificities. *J Ultrasound Med* 1993;12:705–712.

Gordon JD, Hopkins KL, Jeffrey RB, Giudice LC. Adnexal torsion: color Doppler diagnosis and laparoscopic treatment. *Fertil Steril* 1994;61:383–385.

Wilms AB, Schlund JF, Meyer WR. Endovaginal Doppler ultrasound in ovarian torsion: a case series. *Ultrasound Obstet Gynecol* 1995;5:129–132.

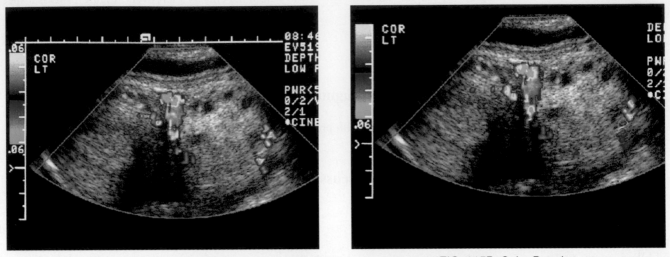

FIG. 115A. Color Doppler.

FIG. 115B. Color Doppler.

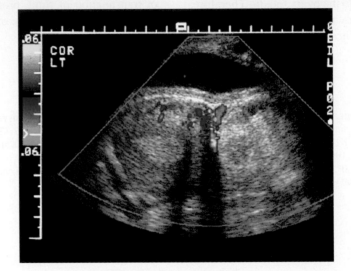

FIG. 115C. Color Doppler.

History

A 19-year-old female with sudden onset of left lower-quadrant pain. Rule out ovarian torsion.

Findings

Figures 115A–C are color Doppler sonograms from an endovaginal study. Note the enlarged left ovary with prominent peripheral follicles. The ovary is increased in echogenicity. There is no intrinsic arterial flow within the enlarged left ovary depicted on color Doppler.

Diagnosis

Left ovarian torsion.

Discussion

Despite the absence of internal flow on endovaginal color Doppler when the left ovary was detorsed at surgery, the ovary was thought to be viable. Therefore, an oophorectomy was not performed. In the past, oophorectomy was routine in all cases of torsion, but more recent surgical practice reevaluates the ovary after detorsing its pedicle, because many ovaries cannot be salvaged. The complete absence of flow in this ovary was strongly suggestive of torsion. However, arterial flow can be preserved in some patients because of the dual blood supply to the ovary. Predicting the viability of the ovary may not be possible with color Doppler imaging. Despite a complete absence of flow on color Doppler, the ovary was viable following detorsion.

References

Fleischer AC, Culinan JA, Kepple DM, Williams LL. Conventional and color Doppler transvaginal sonography of pelvic masses: a comparison of relative histologic specificities. *J Ultrasound Med* 1993;12:705–712.

Gordon JD, Hopkins KL, Jeffrey RB, Giudice LC. Adnexal torsion: color Doppler diagnosis and laparoscopic treatment. *Fertil Steril* 1994;61:383–385.

Wilms AB, Schlund JF, Meyer WR. Endovaginal Doppler ultrasound in ovarian torsion: a case series. *Ultrasound Obstet Gynecol* 1995;5:129–132.

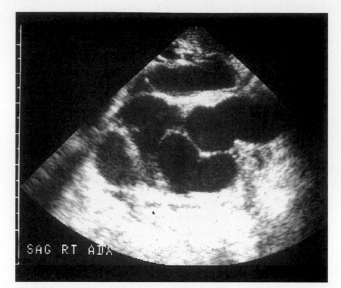

FIG. 116A. Grayscale.

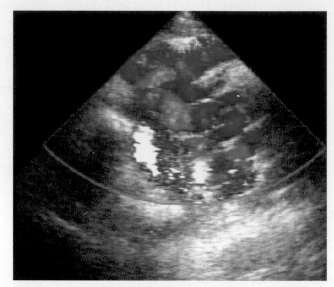

FIG. 116B. Color Doppler.

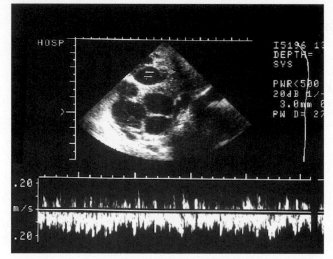

FIG. 116C. Doppler spectrum.

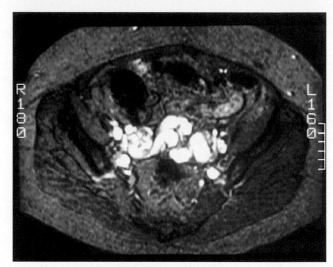

FIG. 116D. GRE MRI.

History

A 49-year-old G6 P6 female with chronic pelvic pain. Rule out adnexal mass.

Findings

Figure 116A is an endovaginal sonogram demonstrating multiple hypoechoic serpiginous structures. Figure 116B is a color Doppler endovaginal sonogram demonstrating that these structures represent blood vessels. Figure 116C, a spectral Doppler tracing, confirms that they are pelvic varices. Figure 116D is a gradient recalled echo, flow-sensitive scan documenting high signal flow in the pelvic varices.

Diagnosis

Pelvic varices as a cause of pelvic congestion syndrome.

Discussion

Varices involving the ovary and broad ligament have been implicated as the cause of chronic pain in pelvic congestion syndrome. Color Doppler sonography can be of significant value in helping to establish this diagnosis and to exclude other adnexal pathology. Both color and spectral Doppler are essential to establish the diagnosis of varices. In some patients, ovarian vein ligation has been used to treat this entity. It is postulated that these varices first develop during pregnancy and, in a small patient, persist post partum. This is usually associated with gross distention of the ovarian vein. In some instances, this may be due to incompetence of the valves within the proximal ovarian vein.

References

Hodgson TJ, Reed MW, Hemingway AP. Case report: the ultrasound and Doppler appearances of pelvic varices. *Clin Radiol* 1991;44:209–219.

Sichalau MJ, Yao JS, Vogelzang RL. Transcatheter embolotherapy for the treatment of pelvic congestion syndrome. *Obstet Gynecol* 1994;83:892–896.

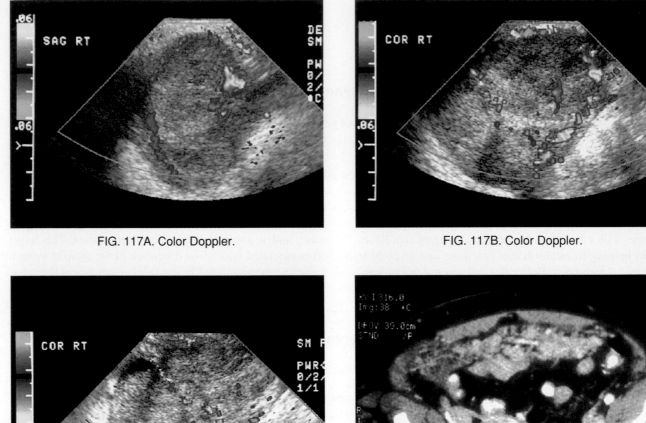

FIG. 117A. Color Doppler.

FIG. 117B. Color Doppler.

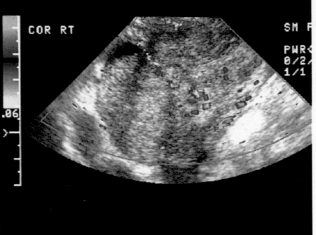

FIG. 117C. Color Doppler.

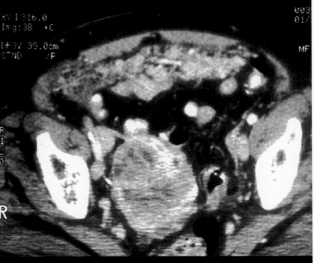

FIG. 117D. Contrast-enhanced CT.

History

A 74-year-old female with a right adnexal mass.

Findings

Figures 117A–C, which are endovaginal color Doppler sonograms of the right adnexa, show a solid mass containing intrinsic color Doppler flow. Figure 117D is a contrast-enhanced CT demonstrating, in addition to the solid right adnexal mass, diffuse infiltration of the omentum.

Diagnosis

Ovarian carcinoma with omental metastasis.

Discussion

The intrinsic color Doppler flow within the adnexal mass clearly established the diagnosis as a solid lesion. The resistive indices were in the range of 0.4 to 0.5, worrisome for malignancy. The main value of color flow is to differentiate a solid lesion from a cystic lesion and to define more clearly the morphologic features that might suggest malignancy. In this patient, CT clearly demonstrated the omental metastases. Color Doppler flow may be particularly useful in evaluating hemorrhagic cysts because these would be entirely avascular. On grayscale imaging alone, they might be confused with solid lesions.

References

Fleischer AC, Rodgers WH, Kepple DM, Williams LL, Jones HW III. Color Doppler sonography of ovarian masses: a multiparameter analysis. *J Ultrasound Med* 1993;12:41–48.

Kurjack A, Zalud I, Alfirevic Z. Evaluation of adnexal masses with transvaginal color ultrasound. *J Ultrasound Med* 1991;10:295–297.

Salem S, White LM, Lai J. Doppler sonography of adnexal masses: the predictive value of the pulsatility index in benign and malignant disease. *AJR* 1994;163:1147–1150.

Stein SM, Laifer-Narin S, Johnson MB, et al. Differentiation of benign and malignant adnexal masses: relative value of gray-scale, color Doppler, and spectral Doppler sonography. *AJR* 1995;164:381–386.

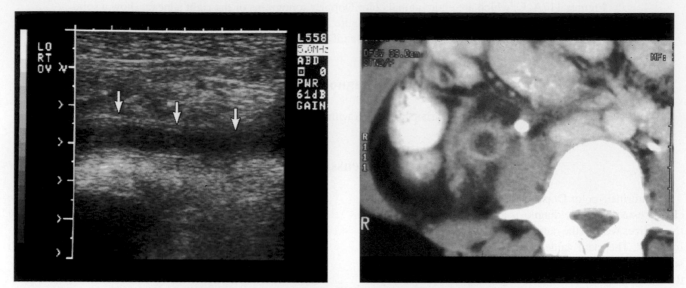

FIG. 118A. Grayscale.

FIG. 118B. Contrast-enhanced CT.

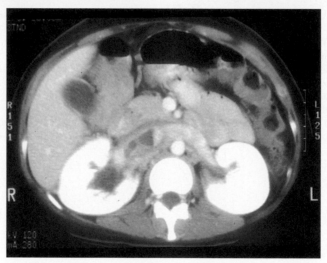

FIG. 118C. Contrast-enhanced CT.

History

A 27-year-old female with right lower-quadrant pain and fever 3 days after a normal vaginal delivery.

Findings

Figure 118A, a longitudinal scan of the midabdomen, demonstrated a tubular noncompressible structure (arrows). Figures 118B and C are contrast-enhanced CTs showing that a thrombus in the right ovarian vein extends into the inferior vena cava.

Diagnosis

Postpartum ovarian vein thrombosis.

Discussion

In postpartum patients, the clinical presentation of right-sided ovarian vein thrombosis may often mimic appendicitis, endometritis, or pyelonephritis. Pain is caused by venous congestion of the ovary. The key to the sonographic diagnosis is recognition of the noncompressible thrombus in the ovarian vein in the right lower quadrant adjacent to the common iliac vessels. Other considerations are a dilated right ureter due to obstruction. Contrast-enhanced CT may also aid in diagnosing this entity.

References

Rooholamini SA, Au AH, Hansen GC, et al. Imaging of pregnancy-related complications. *Radiographics* 1993; 13:753–770.

Witlin AG, Sibai BM. Postpartum ovarian vein thrombosis after vaginal delivery: a report of 11 cases. *Obstet Gynecol* 1995;85:775–780.

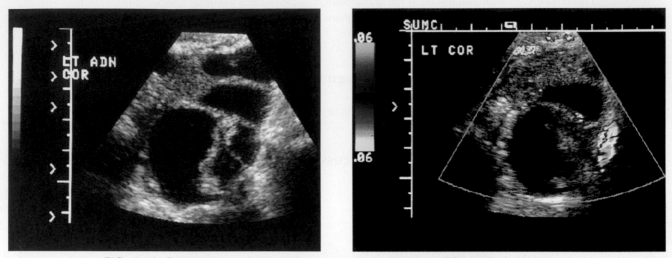

FIG. 119A. Grayscale.

FIG. 119B. Color Doppler.

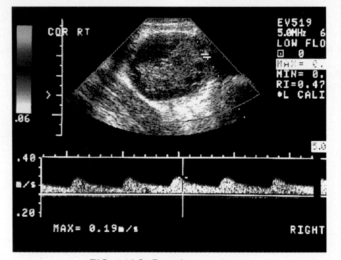

FIG. 119C. Doppler spectrum.

History

A 26-year-old female with right lower-quadrant pain. Rule out appendicitis.

Findings

Figure 119A, an endovaginal grayscale image of the right adnexa, shows a complex cystic mass. In Figs. 119B and C, the internal tissue within the cystic mass is noted to be avascular. Only peripheral flow is detected with spectral Doppler tracings in Fig. 119C.

Diagnosis

Hemorrhagic ovarian cyst.

Discussion

One of the main values of color Doppler sonography with the endovaginal technique is the identification of vascularized tissue within cystic masses. The configuration of the "tissue" within the cyst in Fig. 119B demonstrates straight edges consistent with retracting clot. Hemorrhagic cysts can be confirmed with spin-echo T1-weighted image both with and without fat saturation, which was done in this case (not included). Microscopic hemorrhage is exceedingly rare in ovarian carcinoma, so a demonstration of hemorrhage within a cyst makes it almost certainly benign.

References

Fleischer AC, Rodgers WH, Kepple DM, Williams LL, Jones HW III. Color Doppler sonography of ovarian masses: a multiparameter analysis. *J Ultrasound Med* 1993;12:41–48.

Kurjack A, Zalud I, Alfirevic Z. Evaluation of adnexal masses with transvaginal color ultrasound. *J Ultrasound Med* 1991;10:295–297.

Salem S, White LM, Lai J. Doppler sonography of adnexal masses: the predictive value of the pulsatility index in benign and malignant disease. *AJR* 1994;163:1147–1150.

Stein SM, Laifer-Narin S, Johnson MB, et al. Differentiation of benign and malignant adnexal masses: relative value of gray-scale, color Doppler, and spectral Doppler sonography. *AJR* 1995;164:381–386.

The Testis

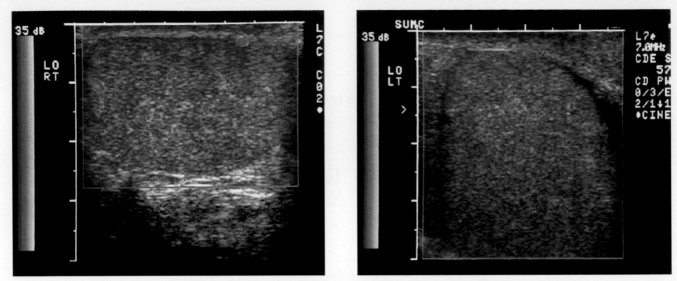

FIG. 120A. Power Doppler.

FIG. 120B. Power Doppler.

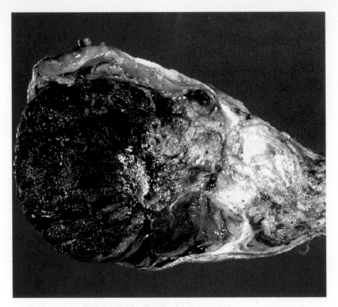

FIG. 120C. Pathology specimen.

HISTORY

A 19-year-old male with a poor response to oral antibiotics for epididymitis, with increased scrotal pain and tenderness over the preceding 48 hours.

Findings

Figure 120A is a sagittal power Doppler sonogram of the normal right testis. Note the clearly identified intrinsic flow within the testis. Figure 120B, a power Doppler sonogram of an enlarged left testis, demonstrates no internal flow within the testis. Figure 120C, a pathologic specimen following orchiectomy, reveals an infarcted testis.

Diagnosis

Testicular infarction secondary to epididymitis.

Discussion

Although relatively uncommon, chronic or severe acute epididymitis may cause testicular infarction by compression and encasement of the testicular artery or vein by an enlarged epididymis. In the vast majority of patients with epididymitis, prompt antibiotic therapy will reduce swelling within the epididymis and spermatic chord, thus minimizing the potential risk of testicular ischemia. Infarction or ischemia may be caused by either arterial or venous occlusion. The color Doppler findings may be indistinguishable from those of acute torsion with absent testicular flow. Some authorities feel that the resultant testicular ischemia may lead to a higher incidence of testicular infection and abscess formation.

References

Flanagan JJ, Fowler RC. Testicular infarction mimicking tumor on scrotal ultrasound: a potential pitfall. *Clin Radiol* 1995;50:49–50.

Kramolowsky EV, Beauchamp RA, Milby WP III. Color Doppler ultrasound for the diagnosis of segmental testicular infarction. *J Urol* 1993;150:972–973.

Rencken RK, du Piessis DJ, de Haas LS. Venous infarction of the testis: a cause of non-response to conservation therapy in epidiymo-orchitis—a case report. *S Afr Med J* 1990;78:337–338.

Vordermark JS, Favila MQ. Testicular necrosis: a preventable complication of epididymitis. *J Urol* 1984;128:1322–1324.

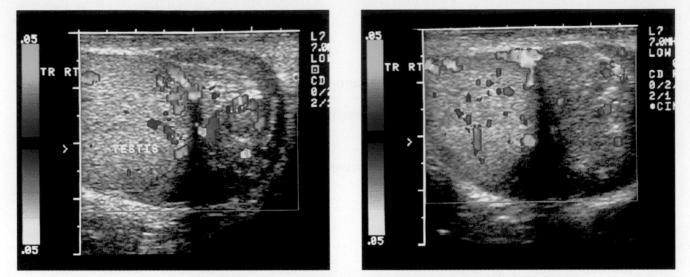

FIG. 121A. Color Doppler.

FIG. 121B. Color Doppler.

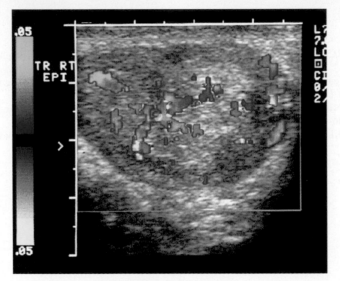

FIG. 121C. Color Doppler.

History

A 5-year-old male with painless scrotal swelling after chemotherapy for leukemia.

Findings

Figures 121A and B are color Doppler sonograms taken in the sagittal plane of an enlarged hemiscrotum. Note the marked enlargement and hypervascularity of the epididymis demonstrated with color flow imaging. Figure 121C, a transverse scan of the epididymis, demonstrates similar findings of hyperemia.

Diagnosis

Leukemic infiltration of the epididymis.

Discussion

Because of a blood–gonadal barrier that limits tissue penetration of chemotherapeutic drugs, the testis is considered a "sanctuary organ." It is therefore not an uncommon site for tumor recurrence of leukemia or lymphoma, much like the central nervous system. Leukemic infiltration of the testis most often presents with painless scrotal swellings, as in this case. Both leukemia and lymphoma may result in focal hypoechoic masses involving the testis or epididymis. The lesions are typically hypervascular when imaged with color Doppler. Based on imaging findings alone, epididymitis or orchitis must be included in the differential diagnosis. From a clinical standpoint, tumor infiltration is generally painless and is generally not confused with acute inflammation.

Reference

Mazzu D, Jeffrey RD Jr, Ralls PW. Lymphoma and leukemia involving the testicles: findings on gray-scale and color Doppler sonography. *AJR* 1995;164:645–647.

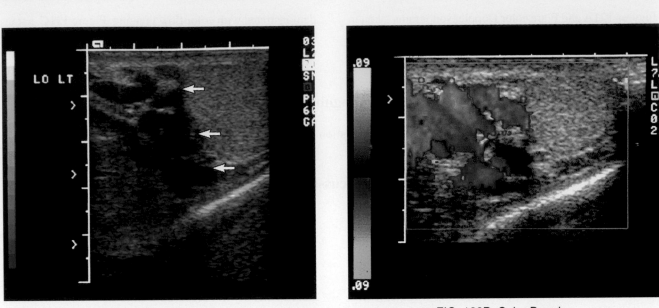

FIG. 122A. Grayscale.

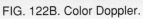

FIG. 122B. Color Doppler.

History

A 35-year-old-male with chronic left scrotal pain. Rule out epididymitis.

Findings

Figure 122A, a longitudinal scan of the left testis, demonstrates normal testicular parenchyma and multiple hypoechoic structures seen adjacent to the testis (arrows). Figure 122B, a color Doppler sonogram obtained during a Valsalva maneuver, shows extensive venous channels representing a large varicocele.

Diagnosis

Left varicocele demonstrated with color flow imaging.

Discussion

Varicoceles may have a variety of clinical presentations, including mild scrotal discomfort and oligospermia. On occasion, varicoceles may be clinically misdiagnosed as either a testicular mass or epididymitis. Color flow imaging can readily establish the diagnosis of varicocele and detect even subclinical lesions that may be important in patients with infertility and low sperm count. Imaging during a Valsalva maneuver is the optimal method for demonstrating flow within the dilated venous structures.

References

Horstman WG, Middleton WD, Melson GL. Scrotal inflammatory disease: color Doppler US findings. *Radiology* 1991;179:55–59.

Horstman WG, Middleton WD, Melson GL, Siegel BA. Color Doppler US of the scrotum. *Radiographics* 1991;11:941–957.

Ralls PW, Jensen MC, Lee KP, Mayekawa DS, Johnson MB, Halls JM. Color Doppler sonography in acute epididymitis and orchitis. *J Clin Ultrasound* 1990;18:383–386.

Wilbert DM, Schaerfe CW, Stern WD, Strohmaier WL, Bichler KH. Evaluation of the acute scrotum by color-coded Doppler ultrasonography. *J Urol* 1993;149:1475–1477.

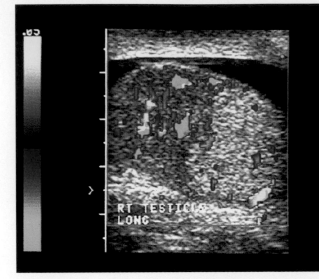

FIG. 123A. Color Doppler.

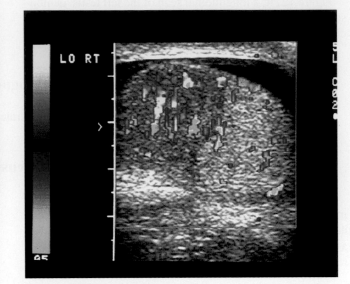

FIG. 123B. Color Doppler.

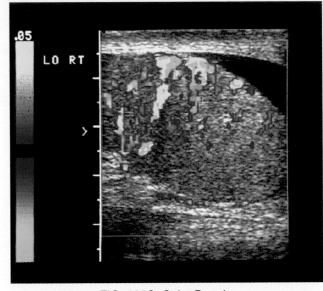

FIG. 123C. Color Doppler.

History

A 19-year-old male with a right scrotal pain. Rule out testicular torsion.

Findings

Figures 123A–C are sagittal color Doppler sonograms of the right testis. Note the small right hydrocele and the marked increased flow in the upper pole of the right testicle. The lower pole of the testicle appears normal in both its echogenicity and color Doppler appearance.

Diagnosis

Focal orchitis mimicking testicular tumor.

Discussion

Orchitis is not often associated with epididymitis. Its extent of involvement may be either focal or diffuse. The grayscale images of the testicle in patients with orchitis may show heterogeneous hypoechoic areas scattered throughout the parenchyma. Involved areas of the testis demonstrate increased flow within the centripetal arteries that is readily detectable with color flow imaging. This patient had focal orchitis in the upper pole of the right testicle. Following a 2-week course of antibiotics, a repeat sonogram showed that the hyperemia had resolved. Follow-up sonography may be indicated in order to exclude a hypervascular tumor, such as a carcinoma or lymphoma.

References

Horstman WG, Middleton WD, Melson GL. Scrotal inflammatory disease: color Doppler US findings. *Radiology* 1991;179:55–59.

Horstman WG, Middleton WD, Melson GL, Siegel BA. Color Doppler US of the scrotum. *Radiographics* 1991; 11:941–957.

Ralls PW, Jensen MC, Lee KP, Mayekawa DS, Johnson MB, Halls JM. Color Doppler sonography in acute epididymitis and orchitis. *J Clin Ultrasound* 1990;18:383–386.

Wilbert DM, Schaerfe CW, Stern WD, Strohmaier WL, Bichler KH. Evaluation of the acute scrotum by color-coded Doppler ultrasonography. *J Urol* 1993;149:1475–1477.

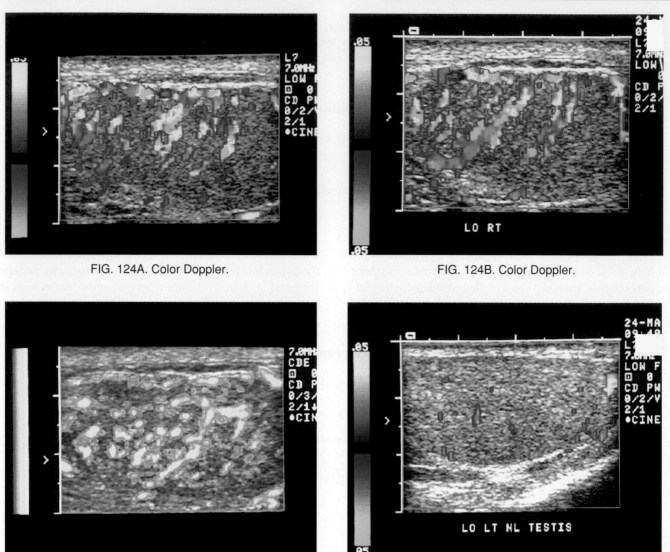

FIG. 124A. Color Doppler.

FIG. 124B. Color Doppler.

FIG. 124C. Power Doppler.

FIG. 124D. Color Doppler.

History

A 22-year-old male with a painful right scrotum. Rule out epididymitis.

Findings

Figures 124A and B are color Doppler sonograms and Fig. 124C is a power Doppler image of the right testis. Note the marked hyperemia and increased flow throughout the entire testis. Figure 124D is a color Doppler sonogram of the normal left testis for comparison.

Diagnosis

Orchitis.

Discussion

Color Doppler sonography is of considerable clinical value in the assessment of patients with acute scrotal pain. Testicular torsion can generally be differentiated from orchitis because of markedly diminished flow. Prominent hyperemia, as noted in this patient, is typical of orchitis. In most patients with torsion, complete absence of flow or marked decrease in flow is evident with color Doppler imaging. Power Doppler imaging improves detection of blood vessels in the pediatric scrotum. In patients with orchitis and focal hypoechoic avascular areas, abscess formation must be considered in the differential diagnosis. Often these patients require hospitalization with administration of intravenous antibiotics because outpatient therapy with oral antibiotics is ineffective. Surgical drainage is required in rare cases.

References

Horstman WG, Middleton WD, Melson GL. Scrotal inflammatory disease: color Doppler US findings. *Radiology* 1991;179:55–59.

Horstman WG, Middleton WD, Melson GL, Siegel BA. Color Doppler US of the scrotum. *Radiographics* 1991; 11:941–957.

Ralls PW, Jensen MC, Lee KP, Mayekawa DS, Johnson MB, Halls JM. Color Doppler sonography in acute epididymitis and orchitis. *J Clin Ultrasound* 1990;18:383–386.

Wilbert DM, Schaerfe CW, Stern WD, Strohmaier WL, Bichler KH. Evaluation of the acute scrotum by color-coded Doppler ultrasonography. *J Urol* 1993;149:1475–1477.

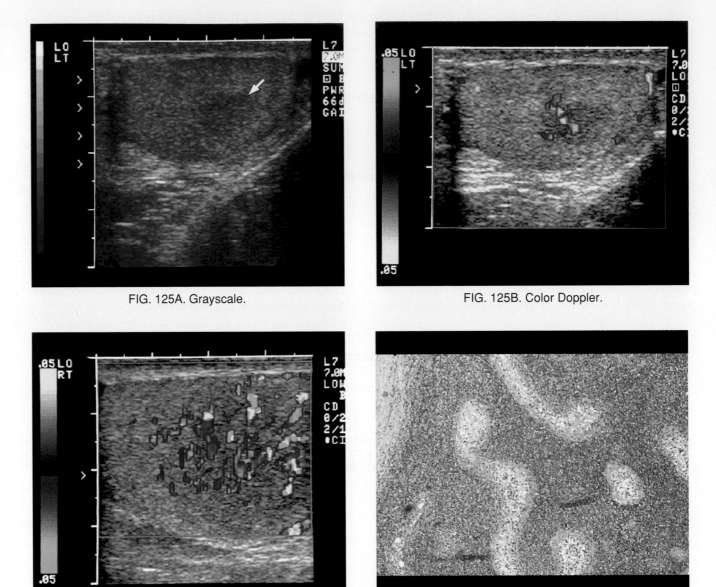

FIG. 125A. Grayscale.

FIG. 125B. Color Doppler.

FIG. 125C. Color Doppler.

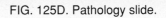

FIG. 125D. Pathology slide.

History

A patient with known lymphoma who had painless scrotal swelling.

Findings

Figure 125A, a sagittal scan of the left testis, shows a small hypoechoic mass (arrow). Figure 125B is a color Doppler sonogram demonstrating that the mass has increased flow compared with the background testicular parenchyma. Figure 125C, a color Doppler sonogram of the enlarged right testis, reveals a hypervascular mass in the lower pole of the right testis. Figure 125D, a slide from the light microscopy from the pathology following right orchiectomy, demonstrates that the focal mass represents non-Hodgkin's lymphoma.

Diagnosis

Bilateral non-Hodgkin's lymphoma of the testes.

Discussion

The small left testicular mass in this patient was nonpalpable. However, the bilateral masses that were hypervascular compared with the normal testicular parenchyma suggested the diagnosis of non-Hodgkin's lymphoma. The palpable mass in the right testis was also hypervascular with color Doppler sonography, which is typical for lymphoma. Thus, lymphoma must be included in the differential diagnosis of focally increased area of flow, such as focal orchitis, which may mimic neoplasm. Compared with patients with testicular tumors, the clinical presentation is generally different in patients with orchitis, because of the presence of pain and fever. This patient had a nontender solid palpable mass and a history of non-Hodgkin's lymphoma. He had been treated with chemotherapy, and it was felt that the testes were the only site of residual disease. This is not infrequent with either lymphoma or leukemia, because the ovaries and testes are considered to be "sanctuary" organs that may harbor microscopic disease that does not respond to conventional chemotherapy.

Reference

Mazzu D, Jeffrey RB Jr, Ralls PW. Lymphoma and leukemia involving the testicles: findings on gray-scale and color Doppler sonography. *AJR* 1995;164:645–647.

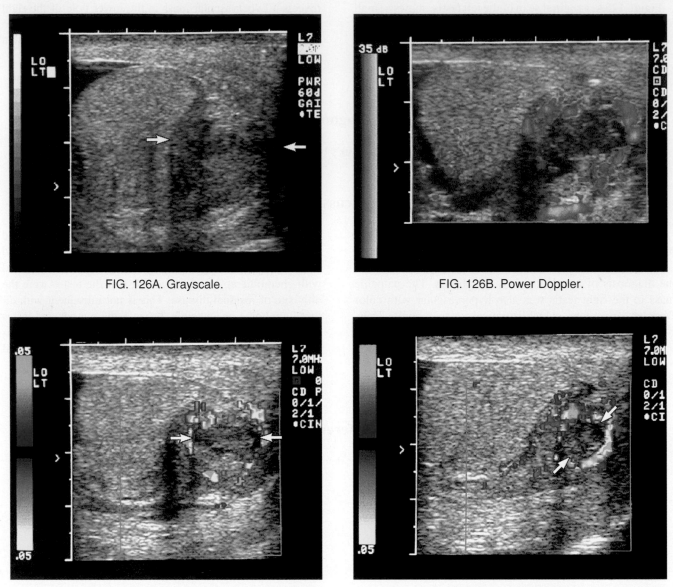

FIG. 126A. Grayscale.

FIG. 126B. Power Doppler.

FIG. 126C. Color Doppler.

FIG. 126D. Color Doppler.

HISTORY

A 22-year-old male with epididymitis not clinically responding to oral antibiotics.

Findings

Figure 126A, a grayscale sonogram of the scrotum, shows marked hypertrophy of the tail of the epididymis (arrows). Figure 126B is a power Doppler sonogram and Figs. 126C and D are color Doppler sonograms demonstrating marked hyperemia of the epididymis with displacement of vasculature around a hypoechoic mass (arrows).

Diagnosis

Epididymitis with early abscess formation.

Discussion

This patient's condition failed to respond to oral antibiotics, and he required hospitalization with intravenous antibiotic administration in the epididymis for 5 days to control the infection. The vascular displacement around a hypoechoic mass suggested early abscess formation. The mass itself was avascular because of liquefied pus. In some patients, surgical drainage is required if fever and sepsis continue despite appropriate antibiotic coverage.

References

Flanagan JJ, Fowler RC. Testicular infarction mimicking tumor on scrotal ultrasound: a potential pitfall. *Clin Radiol* 1995;50:49–50.

Kramolowsky EV, Beauchamp RA, Milby WP III. Color Doppler ultrasound for the diagnosis of segmental testicular infarction. *J Urol* 1993;150:972–973.

Rencken RK, du Plessis DJ, de Haas LS. Venous infarction of the testis: a cause of non-response to conservation therapy in epidiymo-orchitis—a case report. *S Afr Med J* 1990;78:337–338.

Vordermark JS, Favila MQ. Testicular necrosis: a preventable complication of epididymitis. *J Urol* 1984;128:1322–1324.

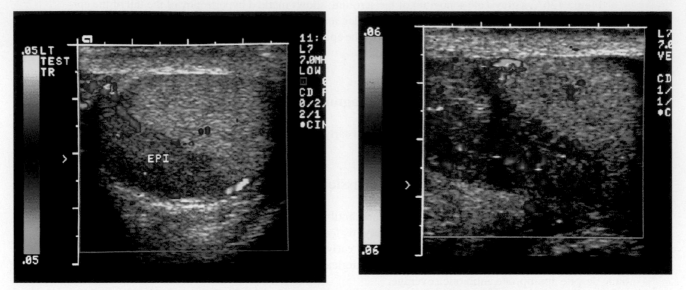

FIG. 127A. Color Doppler.   FIG. 127B. Color Doppler.

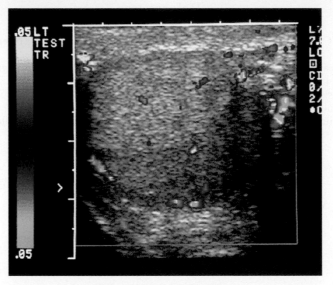

FIG. 127C. Color Doppler.

History

A 19-year-old male with acute left scrotal pain. Rule out testicular torsion.

Findings

Figures 127A–C are color Doppler sonograms of the left testis. Note the marked enlargement of the epididymis, which is diffusely hypoechoic. The color Doppler images demonstrate significant hyperemia of the epididymis, but no associated orchitis.

Diagnosis

Acute epididymitis.

Discussion

Color Doppler sonography may play a pivotal role in the assessment of patients with acute scrotal pain. Often it is very difficult to examine these patients clinically because of severe discomfort. Color Doppler sonography can distinguish torsion from epididymitis, as in this case, with a high degree of confidence. In some patients with early epididymitis, only the tail of the epididymis at the lower pole of the testis is enlarged, which suggests a testicular tumor. Color Doppler sonography is also useful to evaluate complications of epididymitis, such as testicular infarction or abscess formation.

References

Flanagan JJ, Fowler RC. Testicular infarction mimicking tumor on scrotal ultrasound: a potential pitfall. *Clin Radiol* 1995;50:49–50.

Kramolowsky EV, Beauchamp RA, Milby WP III. Color Doppler ultrasound for the diagnosis of segmental testicular infarction. *J Urol* 1993;150:972–973.

Rencken RK, du Piessis DJ, de Haas LS. Venous infarction of the testis: a cause of non-response to conservation therapy in epidiymo-orchitis—a case report. *S Afr Med J* 1990;78:337–338.

Vordermark JS, Favila MQ. Testicular necrosis: a preventable complication of epididymitis. *J Urol* 1984; 128:1322–1324.

SECTION 9

Small Parts

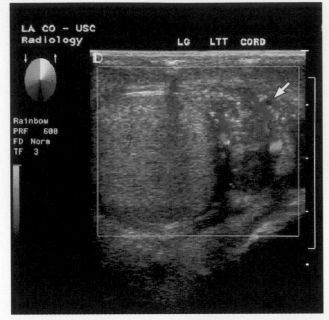

FIG. 128A. Color Doppler.

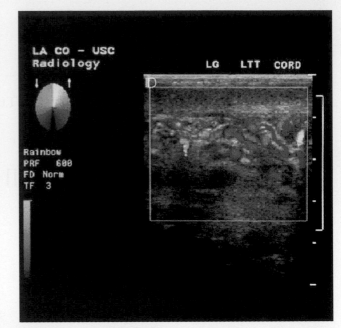

FIG. 128B. Color Doppler.

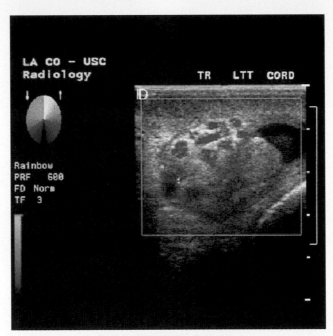

FIG. 128C. Color Doppler.

History

A male; history unknown.

Findings

Figure 128A, a transverse color Doppler sonogram of the left hemiscrotum, reveals normal testicular flow with slightly increased flow in the epididymis (arrow). In most patients, little epididymal flow is identified. Figure 128B is a longitudinal color Doppler sonogram showing increased flow in the vessels of the spermatic cord. Note the intertwined vessels surrounded by and contained within areas of increased echogenicity. Figure 128C, a color Doppler sonogram, reveals flow in an enlarged echogenic spermatic cord. A small hydrocele is noted lateral to the spermatic cord.

Diagnosis

Subacute and chronic epididymitis: echogenic spermatic cord.

Discussion

Color Doppler sonography is an extremely effective technique for identifying and diagnosing inflammatory conditions of the scrotum, especially epididymitis and orchitis. Acute inflammation engenders significantly increased flow in the epididymis or, with epididymitis/orchitis, both the epididymis and testis. Subacute and chronic infections may lead to an enlarged echogenic spermatic cord, as in this case. This patient had subacute epididymitis manifest as increased epididymal flow (Fig. 128A). The spermatic cord hyperechogenicity was strongly suggestive of chronic infection.

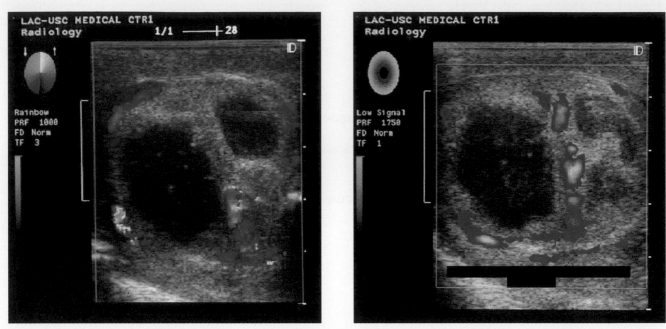

FIG. 129A. Color Doppler.

FIG. 129B. Power Doppler.

History

A 32-year-old male noted pain and swelling of the right hemiscrotum. Without seeking medical assistance, he treated himself with oral ampicillin and chloramphenicol. The symptoms initially subsided, but after 7 days the pain, swelling, and fever became worse. He sought aid at the hospital 3 days later. Because of the scrotal abnormalities, sonography was ordered.

Findings

Figure 129A, a color Doppler sonogram of the right testis, reveals a bilobed intratesticular abscess. Note the marked increased flow in the testicular tissue around the infected areas. Figure 129B, a power Doppler sonogram, likewise reveals increased flow around the testicular abscess.

Diagnosis

Partially treated testicular abscess.

Discussion

Occasionally, inflammatory conditions of the epididymis and testis can result in abscess as a complication of epididymitis and orchitis. Abscesses may occur within the scrotal sac (pyocele) or within the epididymis or testis itself.

Abscesses often occur in the setting of untreated or inadequately treated infection. Despite the potent oral antibiotics, the dosage taken was insufficient to effect a cure.

References

Feld R, Middleton WD. Recent advances in sonography of the testis and scrotum. *Radiol Clin North Am* 1992; 30:1033–1051.

Fobbe F, Heidt P, Hamm B, et al. Improvement in the diagnosis of scrotal diseases using color-coded duplex sonography. *ROFO* 1989;150:629–634.

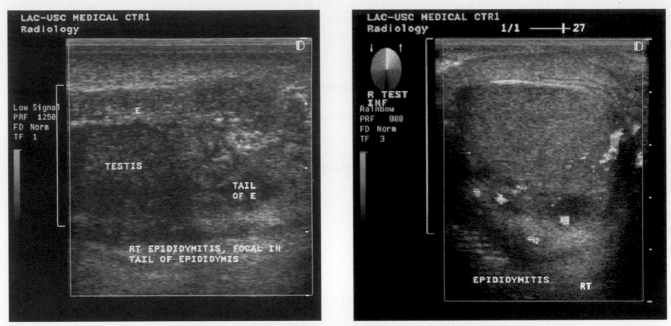

FIG. 130A. Grayscale.

FIG. 130B. Color Doppler.

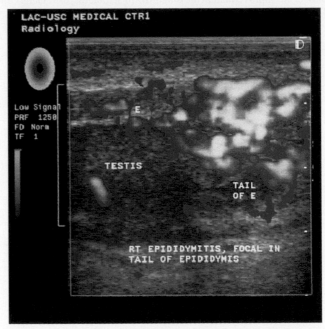

FIG. 130C. Power Doppler.

History

A 28-year-old male with right scrotal pain and a palpable mass in his scrotum, who had a white count of 10,500 and was afebrile.

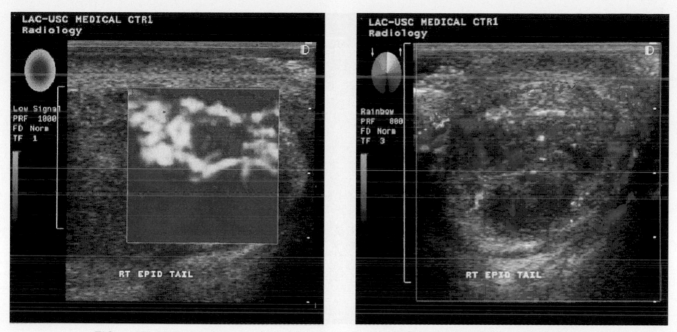

FIG. 130D. Power Doppler. FIG. 130E. Color Doppler.

Findings

Figure 130A, a grayscale sonogram through the lower right hemiscrotum, shows an enlarged body and tail of the epididymis. The epididymal tail is also heterogeneous. The testicle appears normal. Figure 130B, a transverse color Doppler sonogram of the right hemiscrotum, reveals normal flow within the testis. Some scrotal wall thickening is present. There is increased flow within the portion of the epididymis (mainly body). Figure 130C is a power Doppler sonogram demonstrating that the enlarged tail of the epididymis is extremely hy-

peremic, which suggests the diagnosis of focally pronounced epididymitis in the epididymal tail. Figure 130D, another power Doppler sonogram, using a different power map and filtration level, confirms increased flow in the epididymal tail. Figure 130E, a magnified image scanned transversely through the tail of the epididymis, shows internal heterogeneity and areas of increased and decreased flow. This is compatible with epididymitis. The hypoechoic areas with decreased flow may represent areas of infarction or even focal abscess.

Diagnosis

Epididymitis: predominant in tail of the epididymis.

Discussion

Epididymitis and orchitis lead to prominent increased epididymal and testicular blood flow, respectively. Color Doppler sonography displays increased flow on the affected side, especially when compared with the normal contralateral testis and epididymis. In general, the head of the epididymis (near the cephalic portion of the testis) is most severely involved. Diffuse epididymitis with normal testicular flow is also com-

monly seen. Predominant tail involvement in epididymitis, as in this case, is unusual. This patient was treated with intravenous antibiotics for 4 days with nearly complete resolution of symptoms. When discharged, he was to take oral antibiotics. It is impossible to determine whether focal abscesses were present in the enlarged epididymal tail, because conservative treatment was successful.

References

Middleton WD, Siegel BA, Melson GL, et al. Acute scrotal disorders: prospective comparison of color Doppler US and testicular scintigraphy. *Radiology* 1990;177:177–181.

Ralls PW, Jensen MC, Lee KP, et al. Color Doppler sonography in acute epididymitis and orchitis. *J Clin Ultrasound* 1990; 18:383–386.

245

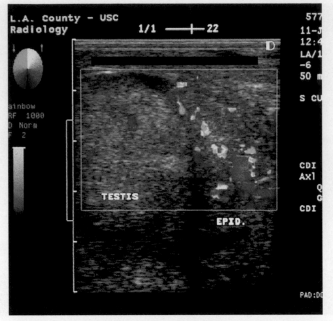

FIG. 131. Color Doppler.

History

A 37-year-old male who was kicked in the groin during an altercation. Scrotal sonography was performed to rule out testicular fracture.

Findings

No testicular fracture is identified in Fig. 131, but the epididymis is enlarged and hyperemic.

Diagnosis

Posttraumatic epididymal hyperemia "traumatic epididymitis."

Discussion

Scrotal sonography in blunt trauma is indicated primarily to determine whether the testis is fractured, because testicular fracture is an indication for exploration. In some patients in whom there is no fracture, posttraumatic hyperemia may result. Epididymal enlargement with hyperemia in this setting is indicative of posttraumatic hyperemia, a finding that has been called traumatic epididymitis. Although the sonographic findings are similar to those found in the usual infectious form of epididymitis, the history is generally sufficient to yield the correct diagnosis.

References

Gordon LM, Stein SM, Ralls PW. Traumatic epididymitis: evaluation with color Doppler sonography. *AJR* 1997 [*in press*].

Lupetin AR, King W, Rich PJ, Lederman RB. The traumatized scrotum. *Radiology* 1983;148:203–207.

Martinez-Pineiro L, Cerezo E, Cozar JM, Avellana JA, Moreno JA, Martinez-Pineiro JA. Value of testicular ultrasound in the evaluation of blunt scrotal trauma without haematocele. *Br J Urol* 1991;69:286–290.

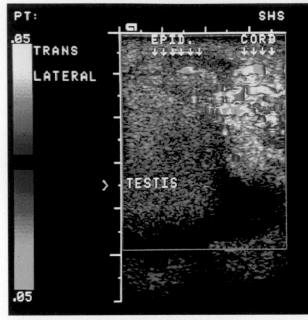

FIG. 132A. Color Doppler.

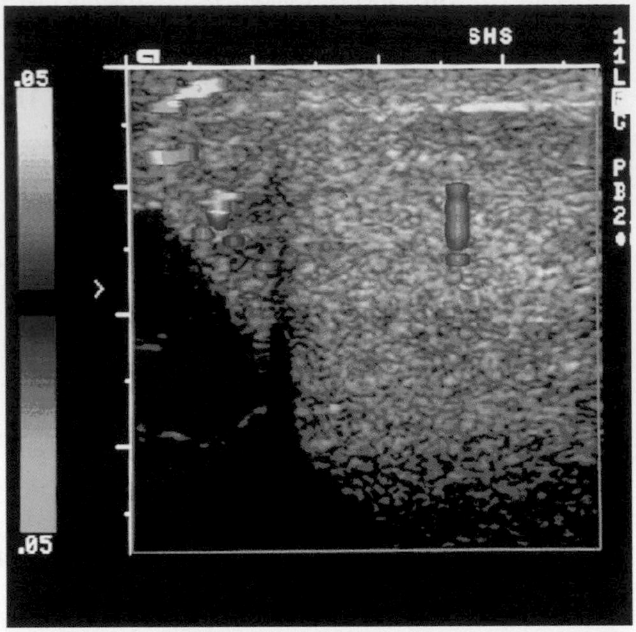

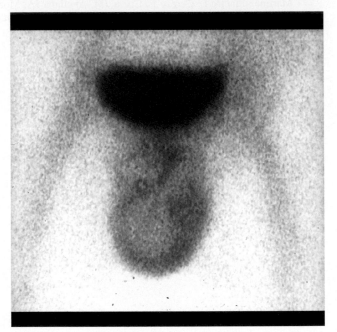

FIG. 132B. Color Doppler.

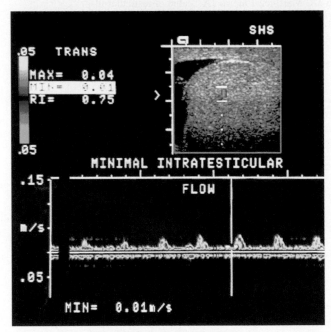

FIG. 132C. Doppler spectrum.

FIG. 132D. Nuclear medicine.

History

A 27-year-old male with acute scrotal pain.

Findings

Figure 132A, a transverse color Doppler sonogram of the left hemiscrotum, shows considerable testicular enlargement and a small associated hydrocele. The epididymis is enlarged and mildly hyperemic. Prominent flow is noted in the spermatic cord. On the left side of Fig. 132B, a color Doppler sonogram of the left hemiscrotum, epididymal hyperemia is noted. A small amount of intratesticular flow is present, less than normally seen. In patients with orchitis, intratesticular color flow is usually markedly increased. Figure 132C, a spectral Doppler of an intratesticular vessel, reveals an arterial waveform, confirming the color Doppler diagnosis of flow. Figure 132D is a nuclear medicine study showing a false-positive "donut" sign. The results of this study were interpreted as diagnostic for testicular torsion.

Diagnosis

Epididymitis/orchitis: testicular ischemia; false-positive nuclear medicine scan for testicular torsion.

Discussion

Absence of flow is a criterion for the diagnosis of testicular torsion. Theoretically, inflammation-related ischemia might lead to absent flow, resulting in an incorrect diagnosis of torsion. Torsion could be diagnosed in a patient who actually had epididymitis/orchitis. Complete absence of flow in the epididymis and testis caused by inflammation must be prohibitively rare, because it has not been reliably reported.

In this patient, there is no diagnostic problem. There is increased epididymal flow, despite decreased testicular flow. Testicular flow is easily identified with color flow sonography and confirmed with spectral Doppler. The nuclear medicine study was insufficiently sensitive to detect the intratesticular flow and the increased epididymal flow. This led to the diagnostic error on the nuclear medicine study.

References

Doherz FJ. Ultrasound of the nonacute scrotum. *Semin Ultrasound CT MR* 1991;12:131–156.

Feld R, Middleton WD. Recent advances in sonography of the testis and scrotum. *Radiol Clin North Am* 1992; 30:1033–1051.

Ralls PW, Larsen D, Johnson MB, Lee KP. Color Doppler sonography of the scrotum. *Semin Ultrasound* 1991; 12:109–114.

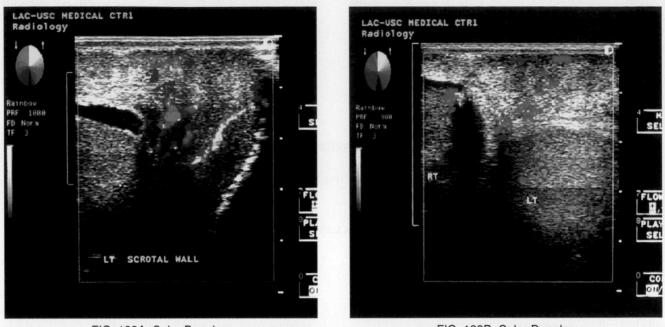

FIG. 133A. Color Doppler.   FIG. 133B. Color Doppler.

History

A 24-year-old male with a 2-week history of scrotal pain and redness.

Findings

Figure 133A, a longitudinal sonogram through the left scrotal wall, reveals marked hyperemia and thickening. A small hydrocele adjacent to the testicle is noted. Figure 133B is a transverse sonogram showing normal testicles bilaterally. The left scrotal wall is much thicker than the right. Note the normal flow within the left testis.

Diagnosis

Scrotal wall thickening and hyperemia from infection.

Discussion

Scrotal wall swelling with hyperemia is commonly associated—but does not always occur—with epididymitis/orchitis. This individual developed a left-sided scrotal cellulitis that involved only the scrotal wall. The right scrotal wall was relatively spared because of the median raphe. The etiology of scrotal wall infection is varied. In extreme cases, emphysematous infections and Fournier's gangrene may occur.

Reference

Lynch PJ. Cutaneous diseases of the external genitalia. In: Walsh PC, Retik AB, Stamey TA, Vaughan ED, eds. *Campbell's urology.* 6th ed. Philadelphia: WB Saunders, 1992:873–875.

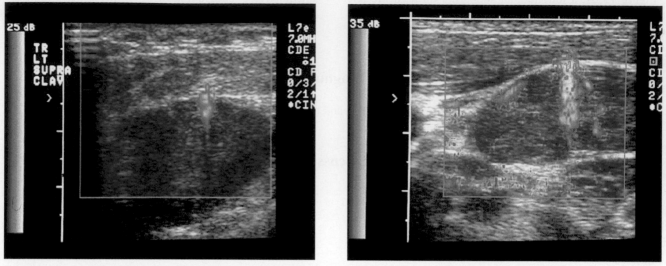

FIG. 134A. Power Doppler.

FIG. 134B. Power Doppler.

History

A 64-year-old female with carcinoma of the breast who developed a left supraclavicular neck mass that was biopsied under ultrasound guidance.

Findings

Figures 134A and B are power Doppler sonograms taken during an ultrasound-guided biopsy of a left supraclavicular mass. In Fig. 134A, note the motion artifact as the needle is oscillated on the surface of the mass. In Fig. 134B, note the power Doppler artifact effect from the tissue oscillation from the needle deep within the mass.

Diagnosis

Power Doppler sonographic guidance for biopsy of supraclavicular lymphadenopathy.

Discussion

One characteristic feature of power Doppler compared with conventional color Doppler is its exquisite sensitivity to motion artifacts. This can be a serious detriment when trying to image the left lobe of the liver, because of cardiac pulsations. Similarly, power Doppler scans of the midabdomen may be degraded in thin patients because of aortic pulsations.

In addition, bowel peristalsis and diaphragmatic motion may also seriously degrade power Doppler image quality. In this patient, however, the "motion artifact" caused by the needle oscillation was extremely valuable in helping to visualize the needle during a percutaneous biopsy.

References

Bude RO, Rubin JM, Adler RS. Power versus conventional color Doppler sonography: comparison in the depiction of normal intrarenal vasculature. *Radiology* 1994;192:777–780.

Newman JS, Adler RS, Bude RO, Rubin JM. Detection of soft-tissue hyperemia: value of power Doppler sonography. *AJR* 1994;163:385–389.

Rubin JM, Bude RO, Carson PL, Bree RL, Adler RS. Power Doppler US: a potentially useful alternative to mean frequency based color Doppler US. *Radiology* 1994;190:853–856.

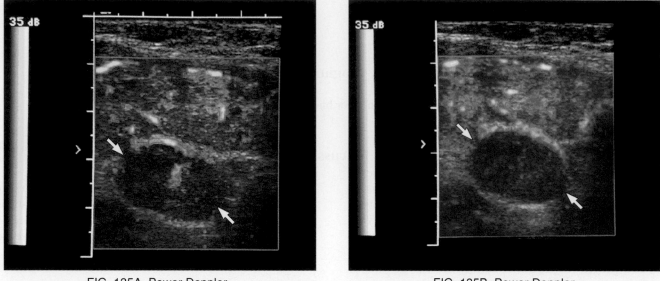

FIG. 135A. Power Doppler.   FIG. 135B. Power Doppler.

History

A 49-year-old male with elevated serum calcium levels. Rule out parathyroid adenoma.

Findings

Figures 135A and B are power Doppler sonograms of the left neck that demonstrate a hypoechoic mass (arrows) with both peripheral and intrinsic vascularity. The mass appears extrinsic to the thyroid and is thus consistent with parathyroid adenoma.

Diagnosis

Parathyroid adenoma.

Discussion

Color Doppler sonography plays a rather limited role in the diagnosis of parathyroid adenomas, which are usually identified with grayscale imaging alone. In general, parathyroid adenomas are less vascular than thyroid adenomas and often have capsular vessels, as in this case. Occasionally, it may be difficult to distinguish a cervical lymph node from a parathyroid adenoma on grayscale imaging. Benign lymph nodes may demonstrate an echogenic fatty hilum with a central feeding artery. Vascularity on the periphery of lymph nodes is relatively uncommon and is useful in diagnosing a parathyroid adenoma.

Reference

Wolf RJ, Cronan JJ, Monchik JM. Color Doppler sonography: an adjunctive technique in assessment of parathyroid adenomas. *J Ultrasound Med* 1994;13:303–308.

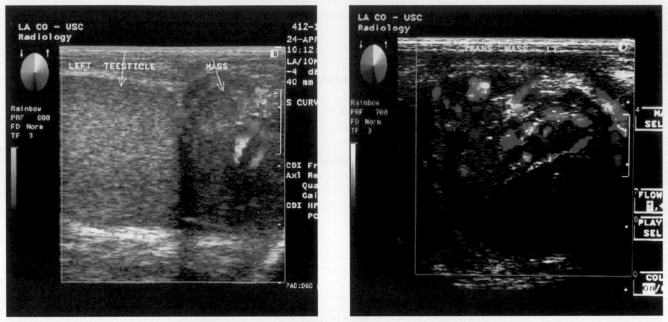

FIG. 136A. Color Doppler.

FIG. 136B. Color Doppler.

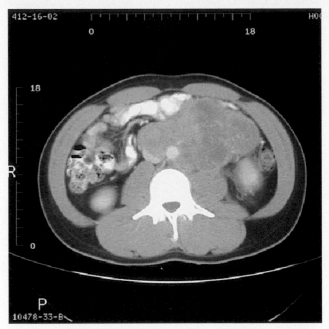

FIG. 136C. Contrast-enhanced CT.

History

A 36-year-old male who came to the Urology Service because of a left scrotal mass. Scrotal sonography was ordered.

Findings

Figure 136A, a longitudinal sonogram of the left hemi-scrotum, reveals a normal left testicle, but a hypervascular mass involving the contiguous epididymis. Figure 136B, a transverse scan through the epididymal mass, shows that the mass is hypervascular. Figure 136C, a contrast-enhanced CT scan of the abdomen 3 months later, reveals a large retroperitoneal mass. CT of the chest (not shown) at this time demonstrated multiple pulmonary nodules.

Diagnosis

Spindle cell sarcoma of the epididymis.

Discussion

Most nontesticular scrotal tumors (scrotal adnexal tumors) are benign. Tumors such as adenomatoid tumors, leiomyomas, and fibromas are relatively common. Epididymal sarcomas, such as this undifferentiated spindle cell neoplasm, are rare. No specific diagnosis was made sonographically, other than scrotal adnexal tumor. The diagnosis was made pathologically from the orchiectomy specimen. Despite chemotherapy, this patient's disease, manifest as the retroperitoneal lymphadenopathy and pulmonary metastases, progressed rapidly.

Reference

Mostafi FK, Price EB Jr. Tumors of the male genital system. In: *Armed Forces Institute of Pathology atlas of tumor pathology*. 2nd series, fascicle 8. Washington, DC: Armed Forces Institute of Pathology, 1973:143–175.

SECTION 10

The Vascular System

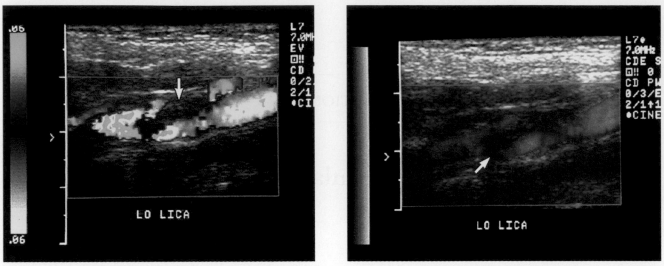

FIG. 137A. Color Doppler.　　　　　　　FIG. 137B. Power Doppler.

History

A 64-year-old male with left hemispheric stroke. Rule out carotid lesion.

Findings

Figure 137A is a sagittal sonogram of the carotid bulb and proximal left internal carotid artery. Figure 137B is a power Doppler sonogram taken at the same level. Note the anechoic filling defect identified on both studies (arrows).

Diagnosis

Left internal carotid artery thrombus.

Discussion

With grayscale imaging alone, it would be virtually impossible to identify this anechoic thrombus. With both color and power Doppler, however, a clearly identifiable intraluminal filling defect consistent with thrombus was evident and was subsequently confirmed with MR angiography. Clot is variable in its echogenicity, depending on its chronicity. Undoubtedly, many anechoic clots are missed with grayscale imaging alone. Unlike intimal plaque, clot may project into the lumen and, in some cases, may be observed to demonstrate transmitted motion with cardiac pulsation. The identification of carotid thrombus was important in clinical management, because this patient was placed immediately on anticoagulation medication.

References

Gardner DJ, Gosink BB, Kallman CE. Internal carotid artery dissections: duplex ultrasound imaging. *J Ultrasound Med* 1991;10:607–614.

Tonizzo M, Fisicaro M, Bussani R, et al. Carotid atherosclerosis: echographic patterns versus histological findings. *Int Angiol* 1994;13:208–214.

Van Damme H, Vivario M. Pathological aspects of carotid plaques: surgical and clinical significance. *Int Angiol* 1993;12:299–311.

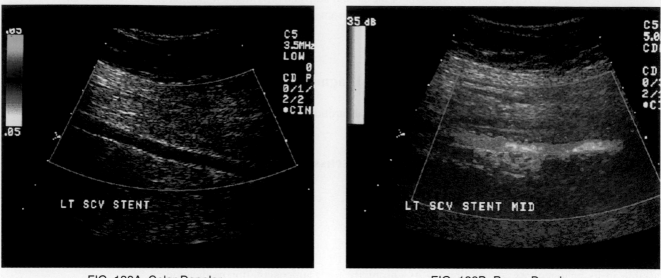

FIG. 138A. Color Doppler.   FIG. 138B. Power Doppler.

History

A 27-year-old male who, after thrombolysis of a superior vena cava clot, had multiple metallic stents placed within the subclavian vein to maintain venous patency. Rule out thrombosis of the stents.

Findings

Figure 138A, a color Doppler sonogram of the left subclavian vein stent, demonstrates no flow within the stent, even using low-volume flow sensitivity parameters. Figure 138B, a power Doppler sonogram of the same stent, clearly demonstrates flow within the stent.

Diagnosis

Vascular patency of a subclavian stent demonstrated with power Doppler.

Discussion

The standard color Doppler image failed to demonstrate flow within the stent in this patient because the vessel containing the stent coursed nearly perpendicularly to the plane of the ultrasound beam. The Doppler equation contains, as one of its components, the cosine of the angle of the ultrasound beam. Because the cosine of 90° is 0, no flow will be demonstrated in vessels perpendicular to the ultrasound beam. This *angle dependency* is one of the major limitations of standard color Doppler. Because power Doppler color encodes the entire energy spectrum of the Doppler signal and not just the mean frequency, it is much less angle dependent than standard color Doppler. Therefore, power Doppler may be used to demonstrate flow even when a significant portion of the ultrasound beam is perpendicular to the vessel. Augmentation of the vascular signal may be a very helpful technique for standard conventional color Doppler to demonstrate flow within venous structures. Alternatively, power Doppler can be used whenever there is a questionable area of thrombosis.

References

Bude RO, Rubin JM, Adler RS. Power versus conventional color Doppler sonography: comparison in the depiction of normal intrarenal vasculature. *Radiology* 1994;192:777–780.

Newman JS, Adler RS, Bude RO, Rubin JM. Detection of soft-tissue hyperemia: value of power Doppler sonography. *AJR* 1994;163:385–389.

Rubin JM, Bude RO, Carson PL, Bree RL, Adler RS. Power Doppler US: a potentially useful alternative to mean frequency based color Doppler US. *Radiology* 1994;190:853–856.

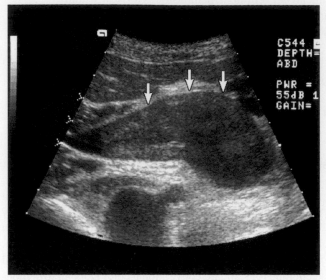

FIG. 139A. Grayscale.

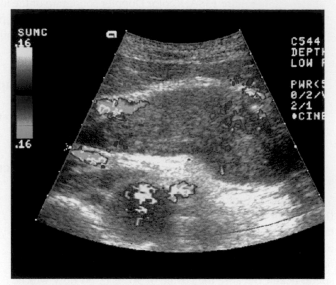

FIG. 139B. Color Doppler.

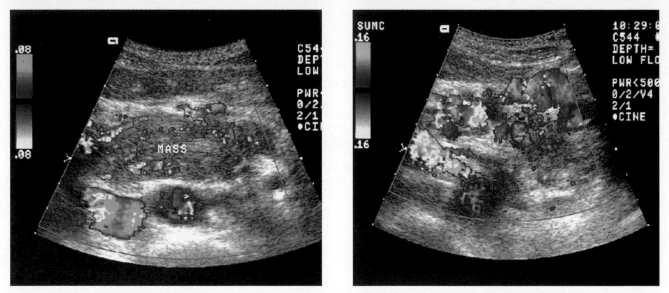

FIG. 139C. Color Doppler.

FIG. 139D. Color Doppler.

History

A 71-year-old male with a palpable mid-epigastric mass 18 months after resection of islet cell tumor of the pancreas. Noncontrast CT scan suggested a recurrent nodal mass.

Findings

Figure 139A, a transverse grayscale image of the splenic vein, shows an enlarged echogenic mass (arrows) entirely contained within the splenic vein. Figures 139B and C are color Doppler sonograms demonstrating intrinsic flow within the mass consistent with tumor neovascularity. Figure 139D is a color Doppler sonogram revealing extensive gastroepiploic and hepatoduodenal collaterals from splenic vein occlusion by the tumor.

Diagnosis

Recurrent islet cell tumor invading the splenic vein.

Discussion

The recurrent tumor in this patient was entirely contained within the splenic vein. The "mass" was therefore not due to adenopathy. It was relatively simple to resect this at surgery because there was no invasion of adjacent tissues. Spectral Doppler tracings (not shown) demonstrated low-impedance arterial flow from the mass. This is diagnostic of tumor neovascularity. The ability to demonstrate with color Doppler the extensive gastric and duodenal collaterals from the splenic vein occlusion was important information that forewarned the surgeon about the need to dissect the hepatoduodenal ligament carefully because of the extensive venous collaterals. Percutaneous biopsy of intravascular tumor thrombus is a safe and effective means of diagnosis. Arterialized flow, however, with a major venous structure is diagnostic of tumor and obviates the need for biopsy.

References

Dusenbery D, Dodd GD III, Carr BI. Percutaneous fine-needle aspiration of portal vein thrombi as a staging technique for hepatocellular carcinoma: cytology findings of 46 patients. *Cancer* 1995;75:2057–2062.

Ralls PW, Johnson MB, Lee KP, Radin DR, Halls J. Color Doppler sonography in hepatocellular carcinoma. *Am J Physiol Imaging* 1991;6:57–61.

Ralls PW, Mack LA. Spectral and color Doppler sonography. *Semin Ultrasound CT MR* 1992;13:355–366.

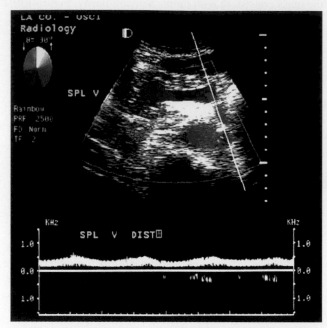

FIG. 140A. Doppler spectrum.

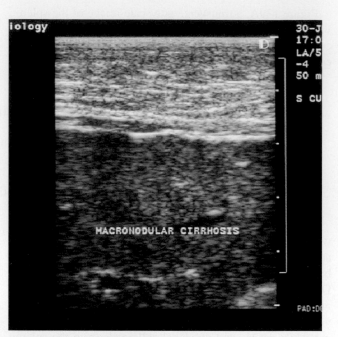

FIG. 140B. Grayscale.

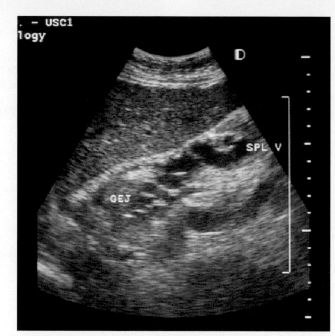

FIG. 140C. Grayscale.

History

A 53-year-old alcoholic female with upper gastrointestinal bleeding. Upper endoscopy revealed isolated gastric varices without esophageal varices. Color Doppler sonography was requested to determine whether splenic vein thrombosis was present.

Findings

Figure 140A is a transverse color Doppler sonogram showing a patent central and midsplenic vein with normal flow on spectral Doppler. Examination of the splenic hilus revealed that the splenic vein was completely open and without evi-

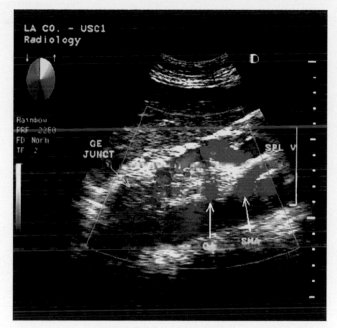

FIG. 140D. Color Doppler.

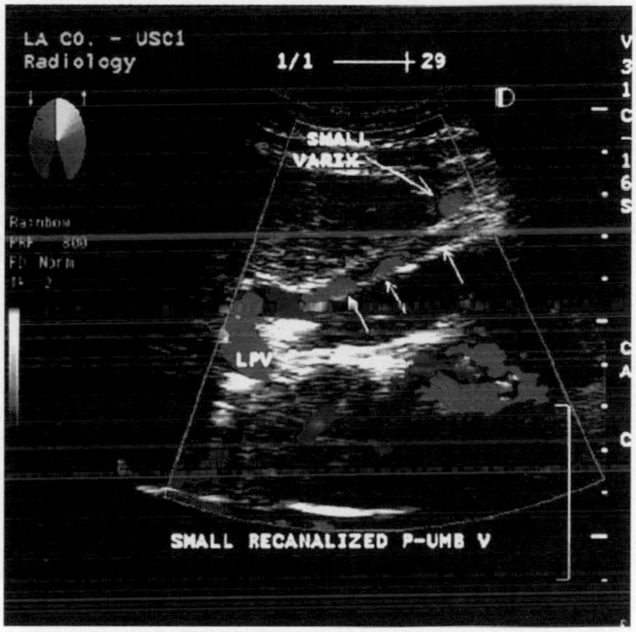

FIG. 140E. Color Doppler.

dence of obstruction. Figure 140B, a high-resolution longitudinal sonogram of the surface of the left lobe of the liver, revealed nodularity compatible with macronodular cirrhosis. Figure 140C, a longitudinal grayscale sonogram of the hepatoduodenal ligament, showed enlarged vessels extending from the region of the splenic vein down to the gastroesophageal junction (GEJ). Figure 140D is a color Doppler sonogram documenting flow in an enlarged, tortuous left gastric (coronary) vein. Varices are seen in the wall of the gastroesophageal junction. Figure 140E, a longitudinal image of the ligamentum teres region, reveals a small recanalized paraumbilical vein with a small associated varix near the tip of the liver.

Diagnosis

Suspected splenic vein thrombosis.

Discussion

Portal hypertension results when venous obstruction occurs in the liver or in the extrahepatic portal veins, and is most often caused by cirrhosis or portal vein clot. Isolated gastric varices are those that occur without concomitant esophageal varices. This finding strongly suggests sinistral (left-sided) portal hypertension caused by obstruction of the splenic vein. Color Doppler sonography is the best examination for determining whether the splenic vein is occluded. Sonographic color flow examination may be difficult, however, because the entire splenic vein is often difficult to visualize. One pitfall is a bridging collateral that simulates a patent vein. Failure to visualize even a small portion of the splenic vein means that splenic vein occlusion cannot be excluded. A short occlusion is sufficient to cause left-sided portal hypertension and gastric varices. In this patient, the splenic vein was open and the endoscopic diagnosis was in error. Subsequent endoscopy confirmed the presence of both gastric and esophageal varices. The most common collateral in portal hypertension related to cirrhosis is enlargement of the left gastric (coronary) vein. The left gastric vein traverses the gastrohepatic ligament (lesser omentum). Generally, blood flows caudally in this vessel and empties into the splenic vein or the proximal portal vein. In this patient, flow was reversed (Fig. 140D) and the left gastric vein was dilated. This type of portosystemic collateral results in esophageal varices. Bleeding from esophageal varices is the most feared complication in portal hypertension because it often results in fatal hemorrhage. Gross varices, such as this, are easy to detect. Smaller left gastric vein varices must be carefully sought in patients with portal hypertension and may be difficult to image sonographically. A careful search of the cephalad margin of the splenic vein with color flow imaging usually suffices.

The presence of a concomitant recanalized paraumbilical vein is somewhat uncommon in a patient with such large left gastric varices. A small varix arising from the recanalized paraumbilical vein often forms at the caudal tip of the liver, as in this case.

Reference

Ralls PW. Color Doppler sonography of the hepatic artery and portal venous system. *AJR* 1990;155:517–525.

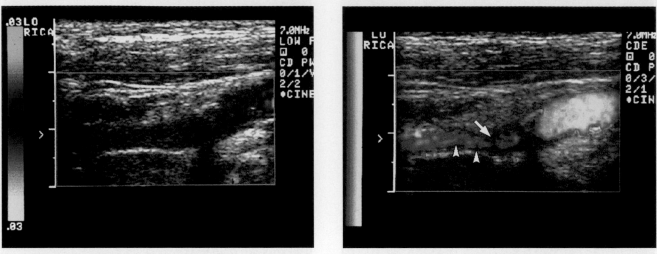

FIG. 141A. Color Doppler. FIG. 141B. Power Doppler.

History

Acute stroke. Rule out right internal carotid occlusion.

Findings

Figure 141A, a color Doppler sonogram of the right internal carotid, demonstrates absent flow, possibly representing a carotid occlusion. Figure 141B is a power Doppler sonogram demonstrating a high-grade obstruction (arrow), but preservation of a small channel of distal flow within the internal carotid (arrowheads).

Diagnosis

High-grade obstruction of the internal carotid demonstrated with power Doppler.

Discussion

The power Doppler findings were of critical importance in avoiding an erroneous diagnosis of carotid artery occlusion in this case. In the setting of total occlusion, carotid endarterectomy is contraindicated. As long as there is any residual lumen, however, carotid endarterectomy may be performed successfully. This patient underwent a carotid endarterectomy following an arteriogram, which confirmed a high-grade stenosis in the internal carotid, but with distal patency. The failure to demonstrate flow with standard color Doppler in the internal carotid may in part be due to its angle dependency. Power Doppler is much less angle dependent than conventional color Doppler. Unlike conventional color Doppler, power Doppler color encodes the entire energy spectrum, not just the mean frequency. When the Doppler angle shifts, the entire spectrum shifts as well, but the area under the curve or the entire energy output of the Doppler signal will not change. Therefore, power Doppler is much less angle dependent and can demonstrate flow even when vessels are perpendicular to the ultrasound beam.

References

De Bray JM, Lhoste P, Dubas F, Emile J, Saumet JL. Ultrasonic features of extracranial carotid dissections: 47 cases studied by angiography. *J Ultrasound Med* 1994;13:659–664.

Mansour MA, Mattos MA, Hood DB, et al. Detection of total occlusion, string sign, and preocclusive stenosis of the internal carotid artery by color-flow duplex scanning. *Am J Surg* 1995;170:154–158.

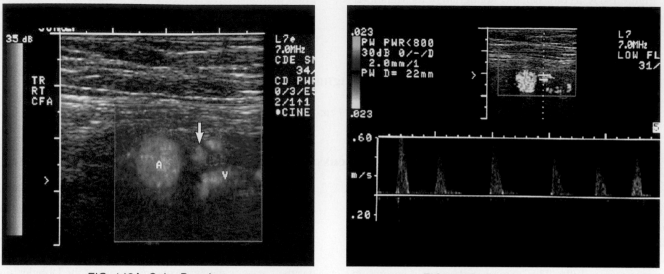

FIG. 142A. Color Doppler.

FIG. 142B. Doppler spectrum.

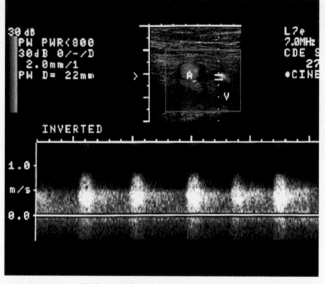

FIG. 142C. Doppler spectrum.

History

A 59-year-old male with right groin bruit 3 days after cardiac catheterization.

Findings

Figure 142A, a power Doppler sonogram of the right groin, shows the right common femoral artery (A) and vein (V). Note the channel of vascular flow connecting the artery and vein (arrow). Figure 142B, a spectral Doppler tracing of this area of flow between the artery and vein, reveals an arterial signal. Figure 142C, a spectral Doppler tracing of the common femoral vein, demonstrates pulsatile venous flow.

Diagnosis

Common femoral artery to common femoral vein arteriovenous fistula following cardiac catheterization.

Discussion

Pseudoaneurysms and arteriovenous fistulas are important but relatively uncommon complications following femoral artery catheterization. They are significantly more likely to occur after coronary balloon angioplasty (3%) than with simple diagnostic cardiac catheterization (0.8%). Often the clinician will feel a palpable thrill over the groin due to the associated turbulence. The actual fistulous tract between the artery and vein was visible with power Doppler imaging, and the transverse view was helpful in identifying this. With standard color Doppler, it is often hard to image in the transverse plane of section due to drop out of signal at 90°. This limitation is not nearly as evident with power Doppler imaging. The sonographic hallmark of an arteriovenous fistula is visualization of pulsatile venous flow and turbulence at the site of the fistula. The natural history of small arterial fistulas suggests that many of these close spontaneously. In fact, this patient's case was followed every other week, and the arteriovenous fistula was closed at 3 weeks. Therefore, surgery should be reserved for the small percentage of patients who demonstrate persistence of the fistula at 3 to 4 months or develop a hemodynamically significant shunt. Power Doppler sonography is an excellent method to follow the status of small arteriovenous fistulas and pseudoaneurysms.

References

Allen BT, Munn JS, Steven SL, et al. Selective non-operative management of pseudoaneurysms and arteriovenous fistulae complicating femoral artery catheterization. *J Cardiovasc Surg* 1992;33:440–447.

Ricci MA, Trevisani GT, Pilcher DB. Vascular complications of cardiac catheterization. *Am J Surg* 1994;167:375–378.

Sidaway AN, Neville RF, Adib H, Curry KM. Femoral arteriovenous fistula following cardiac catheterization: an anatomic explanation. *Cardiovasc Surg* 1993;1:134–137.

Sieunarine K, Ibach G, Prendergast FJ. Femoral arteriovenous fistulas complicating percutaneous cardiac procedures. *Cardiovasc Surg* 1994;2:23–25.

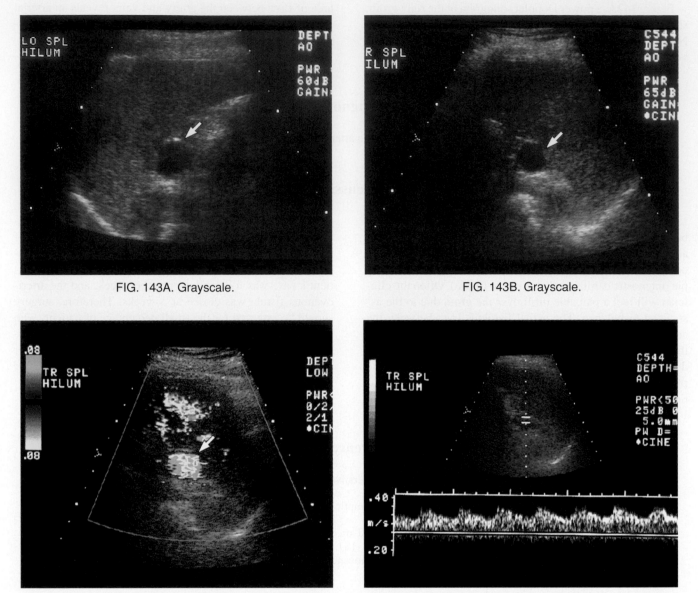

FIG. 143A. Grayscale.

FIG. 143B. Grayscale.

FIG. 143C. Color Doppler.

FIG. 143D. Doppler spectrum.

History

A 70-year-old female with a palpable spleen tip. Rule out splenomegaly.

Findings

Figures 143A and B are longitudinal and transverse scans of the spleen. Note the cystic mass in the region of the splenic hilum (arrow). Figure 143C, a color Doppler sonogram of the cystic mass, demonstrates intrinsic flow within the lesion (arrow). Figure 143D is a spectral Doppler tracing that demonstrates arterial flow within a splenic artery aneurysm.

Diagnosis

Splenic artery aneurysm.

Discussion

Splenic artery aneurysms are most commonly caused by atherosclerotic disease. Splenic artery pseudoaneurysms may be related to pancreatitis, trauma, or interventional procedures. Because they rarely rupture, atherosclerotic aneurysms of <2 cm are generally followed clinically and with imaging studies to ensure stability of size. Once an aneurysm exceeds 2 cm in diameter, however, surgical intervention is indicated because of the potential for exsanguinating hemorrhage. With grayscale imaging alone, this "cystic mass" could have been misconstrued as a pancreatic pseudocyst or possibly a cystic tumor of the tail of the pancreas. Therefore, it is imperative to evaluate all abdominal "cystic masses" with color and spectral Doppler to exclude the possibility of an aneurysm.

References

Huncharek M, Klassen H, Klassen M. Splenic artery aneurysm and upper gastrointestinal bleeding in a nulliparous woman: a case history. *Angiology* 1994;45:733–735.

McDermott VG, Shlansky-Goldberg R, Cope C. Endovascular management of splenic artery aneurysms and pseudoaneurysms. *Cardiovasc Intervent Radiol* 1994;17:179–184.

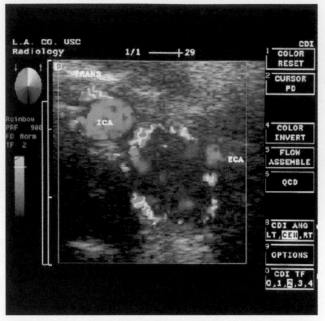

FIG. 144A. Color Doppler.

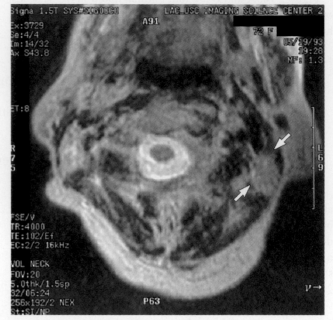

FIG. 144B. T2-weighted MR.

History

A 76-year-old female who was referred for carotid sonography because of atypical neurologic symptoms.

Findings

Figure 144A, a transverse sonogram just above the bifurcation of the common carotid artery, reveals a medium-echogenicity vascular tumor situated between the internal and external carotid arteries. This vascular lesion proved to be a paraganglioma. Figure 144B is an axial T2-weighted MRI. Because of the sonographic findings, an MRI scan of the neck was performed, the results of which were initially interpreted as normal. After the ultrasound was available for comparison with the MRI, a medium-signal-intensity lesion was noted (arrows). This was the carotid body tumor. This is the MRI on which the tumor was most conspicuous. Subsequently, the lesion was removed.

Diagnosis

Carotid body tumor/chemodectoma.

Discussion

Carotid body tumors, or chemodectomas, belong to the group of non-chromaffin-cell paragangliomas. These lesions occur most frequently in patients who are between the ages of 40 and 70, but can be encountered at any age. Chemodectomas generally grow slowly and present as palpable masses. On MRI, these lesions have intermediate signal intensity on all pulse sequences. Flow voids may be seen through the mass. The masses may be inconspicuous, as in this case. Angiographically, carotid body tumors are hypervascular. Derchi et al. showed that sonography can be useful in identifying carotid body tumors and showing internal blood flow. The color Doppler sonography that they performed in two of their 20 patients revealed flow in both instances. Spectral Doppler revealed flow in eight of nine patients. Those authors felt that ultrasound should be the first imaging procedure used in patients with suspected carotid body tumors. A complete survey of the entire neck is needed, however, because bilateral lesions and other cervical chemodectomas may occur.

References

Derchi LE, Serafini G, Rabbia C, et al. Carotid body tumors: US evaluation. *Radiology* 1992;182:457–459.

Gooding GAW. Grayscale ultrasound detection of carotid body tumors. *Radiology* 1979;132:409–410.

Shulak JM, O'Donovan PV, Posture DM, et al. Color flow Doppler of carotid body paraganglioma. *J Ultrasound Med* 1989;8:519–521.

Som PM, Sacher M, Stolman AL, et al. Common tumors of the parapharyngeal space: refined imaging diagnosis. *Radiology* 1988;169:81–85.

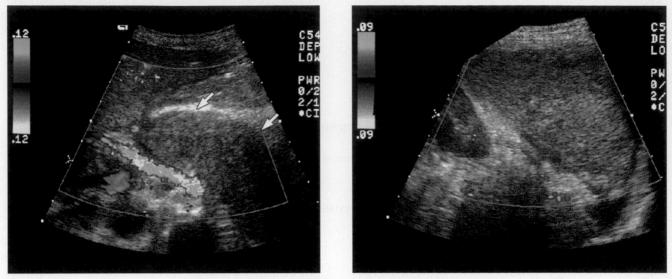

FIG. 145A. Color Doppler.   FIG. 145B. Color Doppler.

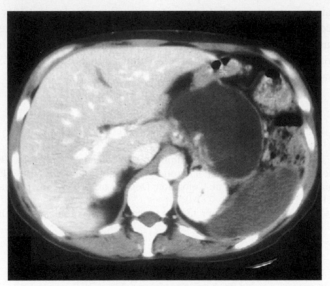

FIG. 145C. Contrast-enhanced CT.

History

A 43-year-old female with endocarditis and severe left upper-quadrant pain.

Findings

Figure 145A, a color Doppler sonogram of the celiac axis, demonstrates a patent hepatic artery but no flow in the splenic artery. Note that the body and tail of the pancreas are enlarged and echogenic (arrow). Figure 145B, a transverse sonogram of the spleen, demonstrates no intrinsic flow within the flow. Figure 145C is a contrast-enhanced CT scan showing infarction of the spleen and extensive pseudocyst formation in the pancreas.

Diagnosis

Arterial embolization to the splenic artery with global splenic infarction and pancreatic pseudocyst formation.

Discussion

This patient proved to have aortic valve endocarditis and subsequent embolization in the splenic artery, which resulted not only in global splenic infarction but also in extensive pancreatic necrosis and pseudocyst formation. The grayscale images of the pancreas and spleen, while not normal, were nonspecific and could be interpreted as hemorrhagic pancreatitis. A definite diagnosis therefore could not be established on the basis of the grayscale images alone. The absence of any intrinsic color Doppler flow to either of these organs strongly suggested the presence of infarction, which was confirmed on subsequent contrast-enhanced CT. The patient ultimately required pancreatic debridement and splenectomy as the pancreatic pseudocyst became infected. The diagnosis of global splenic infarction in this case could be made only with the aid of color Doppler imaging. Segmental splenic infarcts are often peripheral hypoechoic lesions. Global splenic infarction is rare. Even if there is occlusion of the splenic artery, the upper pole of the spleen is usually perfused by the short gastric arteries.

References

Garel C, Hassan M, Legrand I, Magnier S. Contribution of section imaging, echography and MRI, for the diagnosis of splenic infarction in Osler endocarditis: apropos of a case. *Pediatrie* 1990;45:387–390.

Goerg C, Schwerk WB. Splenic infarction: sonographic patterns, diagnosis, follow-up, and complications. *Radiology* 1990;174:803–807.

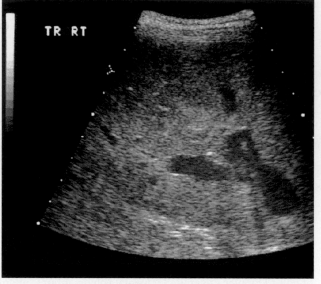

FIG. 146A. Grayscale.

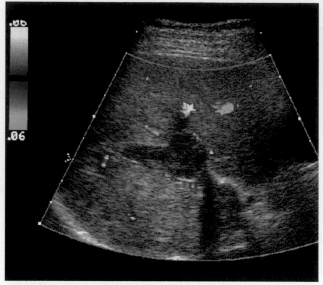

FIG. 146B. Color Doppler.

History

A 29-year-old male with mid-epigastric pain and elevated liver function tests 6 weeks following splenectomy for idiopathic thrombocytopenia.

Findings

Figure 146A, a grayscale sonogram of the porta hepatis, demonstrates increased echogenicity within the portal vein. Figure 146B is a color Doppler sonogram demonstrating no flow within the portal vein. Hepatic arterial flow is seen adjacent to the thrombosed portal vein.

Diagnosis

Portal vein thrombosis secondary to splenectomy.

Discussion

Thrombosis of the portal venous system (particularly of the splenic vein) is a well-known complication of splenectomy. Although the exact reasons are somewhat controversial, predisposing factors include intraoperative surgical trauma, postoperative changes in platelet aggregation, and increased blood viscosity. The overall incidence of splenic vein thrombosis is ~7%. Thrombosis of the splenic portal venous system may be clinically silent and evolve into extrahepatic portal hypertension if anticoagulant therapy is not instituted promptly after diagnosis. It is therefore prudent to evaluate patients following splenectomy with color flow Doppler imaging routinely to diagnose this complication early in the clinical course. The only clinical finding may be slight elevation in the liver function test results.

References

Petit P, Bret PM, Atri M, Hreno A, Casola G, Gianfelice D. Splenic vein thrombosis after splenectomy: frequency and role of imaging. *Radiology* 1994;190:65–68.

Skarsgard E, Doski J, Jaksic T, et al. Thrombosis of the portal venous system after splenectomy for pediatric hematologic disease. *J Pediatr Surg* 1993;28:1109–1112.

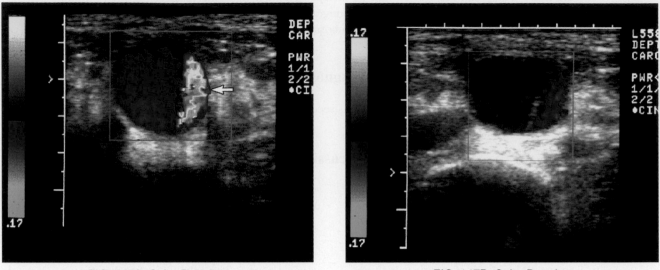

FIG. 147A. Color Doppler.   FIG. 147B. Color Doppler.

History

A 73-year-old male with mid-epigastric pain. Rule out acute pancreatitis.

Findings

Figures 147A and B are transverse color Doppler sonograms of the midabdominal aorta. Note the two distinct flow channels within the abdominal aorta. The true lumen (arrow) is seen laterally and demonstrates high-velocity flow with aliasing. In Fig. 147A, the false lumen is color coded in blue. This image was obtained during systole. In diastole (Fig. 147B), note that flow is absent in the false lumen.

Diagnosis

Abdominal aortic dissection.

Discussion

In most patients with clinically suspected abdominal aortic dissections, either contrast-enhanced CT or MRI is the imaging method of choice. In this case, the diagnosis was confused with pancreatitis, and sonography was performed as a screening study. Most cases of aortic dissection involving the abdominal aorta are extensions from thoracic aortic dissections. In selected cases, however, the dissection may be confined to the abdominal aorta. A "pseudodissection" may be noted with color Doppler imaging in patients with markedly turbulent flow in the aorta. In these cases, no intimal flap is identified, and the turbulent flow is visualized both in systole and in diastole.

References

Conrad MR, Davis GM, Green CE, Curry TS II. Real-time ultrasound in the diagnosis of acute dissecting aneurysms of the abdominal aorta. *AJR* 1979;132:115–116.

Giyanani VL, Krebs CA, Nail LA, Eisenberg RL, Parvey HR. Diagnosis of abdominal aortic dissection by image-directed Doppler sonography. *J Clin Ultrasound* 1989;17:445–448.

Kittredge RD, Gordon RB. CT demonstration of dissecting hematoma originating in abdominal aorta. *J Comput Assist Tomogr* 1987;11:279–281.

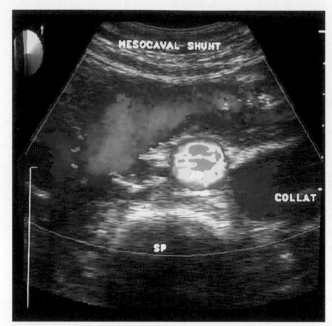

FIG. 148A. Color Doppler.

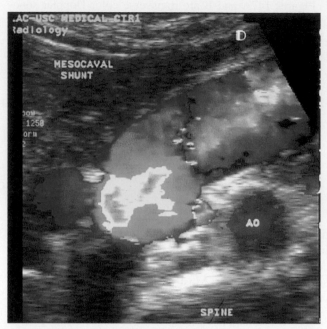

FIG. 148B. Color Doppler.

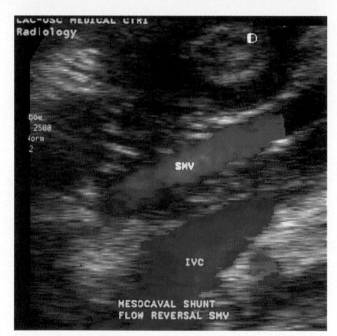

FIG. 148C. Color Doppler.

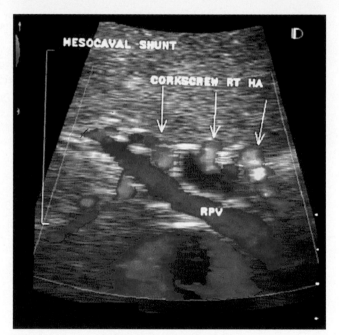

FIG. 148D. Color Doppler.

History

Twenty years earlier, this alcoholic with cirrhosis had several episodes of bleeding from esophageal varices. Because of prominent collaterals in the porta hepatis and hepatoduodenal ligament region, a mesocaval shunt was performed, which anastomosed the peripheral superior mesenteric vein with the inferior vena cava.

Findings

Figure 148A is a transverse color Doppler sonogram in the region of the shunt. Exuberant flow is noted through the shunt between the superior mesenteric vein and the inferior vena cava. The aorta is seen dorsally, just ventral to the spine. A collateral is seen to the left of the abdominal aorta. Figure 148B, an enlarged color Doppler sonogram of the region of the anastomosis between the shunt and the inferior vena cava, reveals marked enlargement of the inferior vena cava (much larger than the aorta) and the large patent shunt. Figure 148C, a longitudinal sonogram of the superior mesenteric vein, shows reversed red-coded, hepatofugal flow within the superior mesenteric vein. Blood is flowing from the liver through the superior mesenteric vein into the decompressing shunt. The mesocaval shunt is caudal to the portion of the superior mesenteric vein. Figure 148D, a transverse sonogram of the intrahepatic right portal vein, shows flow reversal in the right portal vein and its anterior and posterior segmental branches. Prominent arterial flow in the right hepatic artery is identified by its "corkscrew" appearance.

Diagnosis

Mesocaval shunt.

Discussion

Fatal hemorrhage from esophageal varices is the most feared complication of portal hypertension. In this case, a mesocaval shunt was performed to decompress bleeding esophageal varices. The success of the shunt and the patient's success in curtailing his alcohol intake led to a 20-year survival. The shunt decompresses the portal venous system by connecting the distal superior mesenteric vein to the inferior vena cava in an "H"-graft fashion. Although artificial graft materials are currently used, this patient underwent a native vein graft. Successful decompression led to flow reversal in the intrahepatic portal veins, the main portal vein, and the superior mesenteric vein, as demonstrated by these images. Increased arterial flow to the liver, sometimes called *arterialization*, is a homeostatic mechanism to preserve hepatic blood supply. In this case, portal venous blood flow was reversed, resulting in a net negative portal vein blood flow from the liver. More common shunts to compress bleeding esophageal varices include end-to-side portocaval shunts, distal splenorenal shunts, and TIPS procedures.

Reference

Ralls PW. Color Doppler sonography of the hepatic artery and portal venous system. *AJR* 1990;155:517–525.

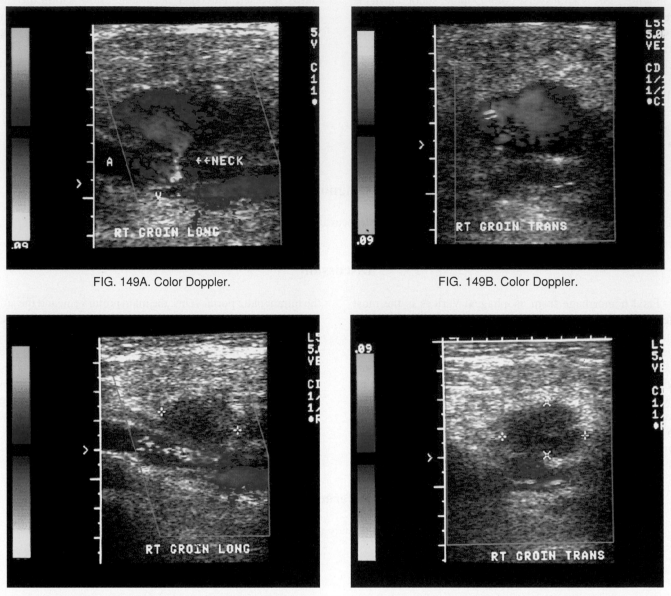

FIG. 149A. Color Doppler.

FIG. 149B. Color Doppler.

FIG. 149C. Color Doppler after compression.

FIG. 149D. Color Doppler after compression.

History

A 64-year-old male with a palpable right groin mass following cardiac catheterization.

Findings

Figures 149A and B are longitudinal and transverse color Doppler sonograms of the right common femoral artery. Note the large pseudoaneurysm anterior to the common femoral artery. Figures 149C and D are scans obtained following 40 minutes of intermittent compression of the neck of the pseudoaneurysm that demonstrate complete thrombosis of the pseudoaneurysm.

Diagnosis

Color Doppler-directed occlusion of femoral artery pseudoaneurysm.

Discussion

Femoral artery pseudoaneurysms are a well-recognized complication of arterial catheterization. This is particularly true following cardiac catheterization because of the large catheters and sheaths that are used, as well the use of anticoagulation with heparin. The use of color Doppler imaging is essential to distinguish an avascular hematoma from a pseudoaneurysm. With color Doppler imaging, compression can be applied directly over the neck of the pseudoaneurysm. It is highly successful for occluding pseudoaneurysms without surgery, but is much less successful in patients who are administered anticoagulants, because clot cannot be created within the pseudoaneurysm. Generally a 10-minute period of compression is applied with the ultrasound transducer, followed by 30 to 60 seconds of noncompression. The flow in the femoral artery is monitored continuously with color Doppler imaging. Generally 30 to 60 minutes of compression is required to occlude the pseudoaneurysm.

References

Coley BD, Roberts AC, Fellmeth BD, Valji K, Bookstein JJ, Hye RJ. Postangiographic femoral artery pseudoaneurysms: further experience in US-guided compression repair. *Radiology* 1995;194:307–311.

Schaub F, Theiss W, Heinz M, Zagel M, Schomig A. New aspects in ultrasound-guided compression repair of postcatheterization femoral artery injuries. *Circulation* 1994;90:1861–1865.

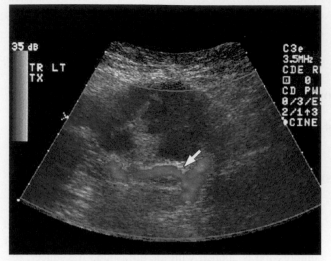

FIG. 150A. Power Doppler.

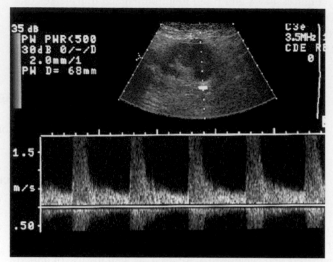

FIG. 150B. Doppler spectrum.

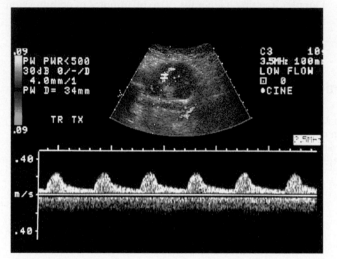

FIG. 150C. Doppler spectrum.

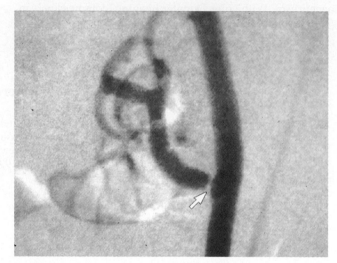

FIG. 150D. Arteriogram.

History

A 44-year-old female with persistent hypertension 2 months following renal transplantation.

Findings

Figure 150A is a power Doppler image of the transplanted renal artery anastomosis (arrow) to the external iliac artery. Figure 150B, a spectral Doppler tracing taken just beyond the anastomosis, demonstrates marked elevation of systolic flow (>200 cm/second). Figure 150C, a spectral Doppler tracing from intrarenal vasculature, demonstrates marked blunting of the waveform. Figure 150D is a selected external iliac arteriogram showing a weblike stenosis (arrow) at the proximal anastomosis of the renal artery.

Diagnosis

Stenosis of renal artery transplant with intrarenal tarvus–parvus waveform.

Discussion

Power Doppler was very helpful in locating the region of the anastomosis between the transplant renal artery and the external iliac artery. Spectral Doppler tracings, however, were required to demonstrate the extremely high velocities from the flow jet caused by the tight stenosis at the anastomosis. Downstream from the stenosis, intrarenal vessels demonstrated the typical tarvus–parvus waveform characterized by a slow upstroke and blunted amplitude. At angiography, a 40-mm gradient was noted across this tight "irislike" stenosis. This was successfully angioplastied and, although the patient's blood pressure did not return to normal, her hypertension was readily controlled with medication. In general, a velocity of >200 cm/second indicates hemodynamically significant stenoses at the anastomosis of the renal and external iliac arteries. Immediately after transplantation, transiently increased velocity may be measured at the arterial anastamosis. This generally normalizes in several weeks. Certainly at 2 months, as in this case, velocity measurements of >200 cm/second taken at the level of anastamosis indicate a functionally significant stenosis. Many of these stenoses can be successfully treated with angioplasty.

References

Plainfosse MC, Calonge VM, Beyloune-Mainardi C, Glotz D, Duboust A. Vascular complications in the adult kidney transplant recipient. *J Clin Ultrasound* 1992;20:517–527.

Tublin ME, Dodd GD III. Sonography of renal transplantation. *Radiol Clin North Am* 1995;33:447–459.

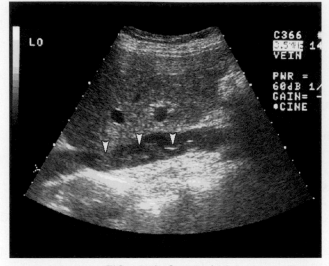

FIG. 151A. Grayscale.

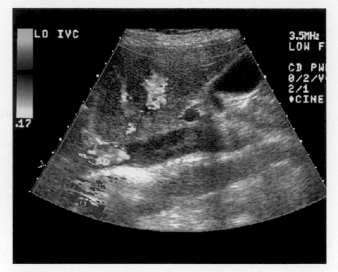

FIG. 151B. Color Doppler.

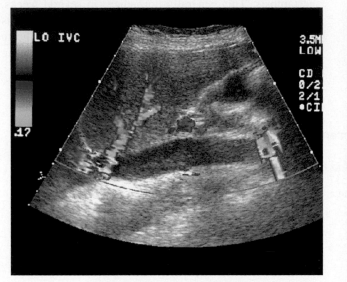

FIG. 151C. Color Doppler.

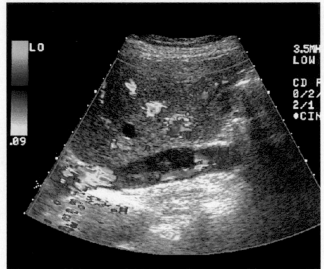

FIG. 151D. Color Doppler.

History

Carcinoma of the lung with vague upper abdominal pain. Rule out liver metastases.

Findings

Figure 151A, a grayscale image of the inferior vena cava, demonstrates internal low-level echoes (arrowheads). Figures 151B–D are sagittal color Doppler sonograms showing extensive thrombus in the inferior vena cava.

Diagnosis

Acute thrombosis of the inferior vena cava.

Discussion

With grayscale imaging alone, the subtle thrombus in the inferior vena cava in this patient was quite hypoechoic and difficult to identify. Color Doppler imaging was extremely valuable in confirming thrombus within the inferior vena cava. The etiology of the inferior vena caval clot, though uncertain, was likely related to a hypercoagulable state associated with a paraneoplastic syndrome caused by the patient's underlying lung carcinoma. This patient was aggressively treated with anticoagulation therapy and did not develop clinically apparent pulmonary emboli sequela. This case underscores that all questionable grayscale abnormalities of the vascular system should be carefully evaluated with color Doppler in order not to miss such clinically important findings as inferior vena caval thrombosis.

References

Hubsch P, Schurawitzki H, Susani M, et al. Color Doppler imaging of inferior vena cava: identification of tumor thrombus. *J Ultrasound Med* 1992;11:639–645.

Lim JH, Park JH, Auh YH. Membranous obstruction of the inferior vena cava: comparison of findings at sonography, CT and venography. *AJR* 1992;159:515–520.

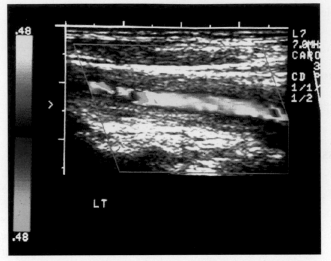

FIG. 152A. Color Doppler.

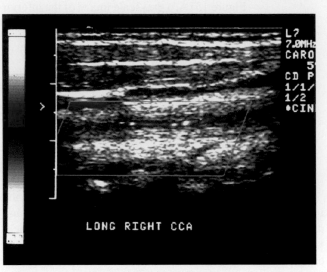

FIG. 152B. Color Doppler.

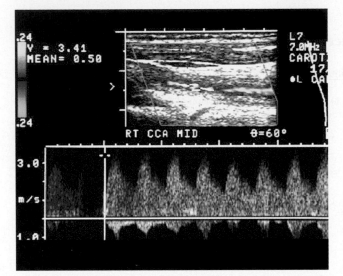

FIG. 152C. Doppler spectrum.

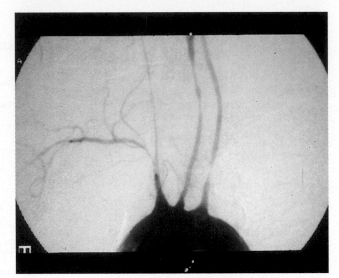

FIG. 152D. Arteriogram.

History

A 15-year-old female with left hemispheric stroke.

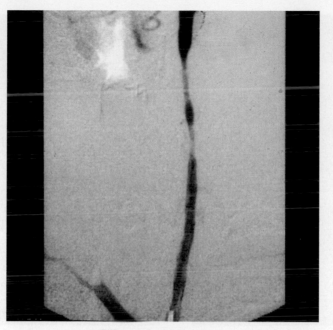

FIG. 152E. Arteriogram.

Findings

Figure 152A, a longitudinal color Doppler sonogram of the left carotid, shows marked intimal and mural thickening. Figure 152B demonstrates marked narrowing of the right carotid artery as well. Note the high velocities within the right common carotid artery consistent with a high-grade stenosis (Fig. 152C). Figure 152D is an arch arteriogram demonstrating marked narrowing of the great vessels consistent with Takayasu's aortitis. Figure 152E is a selective right carotid injection also demonstrating marked luminal narrowing.

Diagnosis

Takayasu's aortitis involving the carotid artery.

Discussion

Stroke is rare in young individuals without trauma or vascular malformations. The marked mural thickening of the common carotids in this patient was caused by Takayasu's arteritis, which was subsequently confirmed at biopsy. The diffuse symmetric intimal thickening of the vessels in this case is typical of vasculitis rather than atherosclerosis.

References

Jorens PG, Williame LM, Tombeur JP, Kockx MM, Parizel GA, Zeyen TG. Takayasu's disease and atherosclerosis. *J Cardiovasc Surg* 1991;32:373–375.

Sato R, Sato Y, Ishikawa H, et al. Takayasu's disease associated with ulcerative colitis. *Intern Med* 1994; 33:759–763.

Sawada S, Tanigawa N, Kobayashi M, et al. Treatment of Takayasu's aortitis with self-expanding metallic stents (Gianturco stents) in two patients. *Cardiovasc Intervent Radiol* 1994;17:102–105.

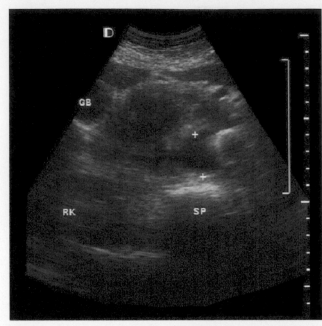

FIG. 153A. Grayscale.

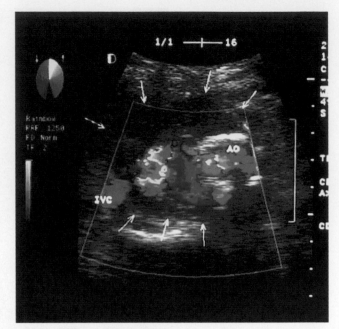

FIG. 153B. Color Doppler.

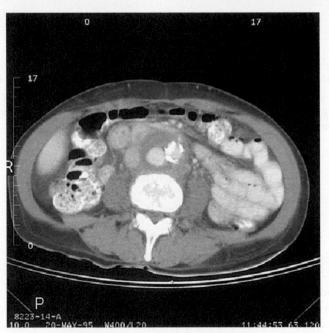

FIG. 153C. Contrast-enhanced CT.

History

A 56-year-old male intravenous drug user with lower abdominal pain and fever. A pulsatile mass was palpated.

Findings

Figure 153A is a transverse grayscale sonogram revealing a large hematoma surrounding a calcified distal abdominal aorta, just above the level of the aortic bifurcation. A central anechoic mass is noted to the right of the distal aorta. Figure 153B is a transverse color Doppler sonogram showing that this mass is a pseudoaneurysm arising from the distal abdominal aorta. The hypoechoic hematoma (arrows) is noted around the pseudoaneurysm. Figure 153C is a contrast-enhanced CT scan confirming the sonographic findings; vascular contrast opacifies the pseudoaneurysm.

Diagnosis

Mycotic aneurysm abdominal aorta.

Discussion

Mycotic pseudoaneurysms have a propensity to occur at, or near, bifurcations or vascular malformations. This lesion appeared just cephalad to the bifurcation of the abdominal aorta. Intravenous drug users are especially susceptible to mycotic aneurysms. Endocarditis is often the antecedent condition. About two-thirds of mycotic aneurysms occur in the femoral arteries, with the aorta the next most common site (~10%). Mycotic aneurysms are less common since the advent of effective heart valve surgery to replace infected valves.

Reference

Reddy DJ, Ernst CB. Infected aneurysms. In: Rutherford RB, ed. *Vascular surgery*. 4th ed. Philadelphia: WB Saunders, 1995:1140–1141.

SUBJECT INDEX

Subject Index

Page references followed by *f* or *t* indicate figures or tables, respectively.

A

Abdominal aorta
  dissection, 280*f*, 280–281
  flow display with lower frequency, 10, 10*f*
  mycotic aneurysm, 292*f*, 292–293
  pseudodissection, 281
Abdominal cystic masses, 157, 273
Abscesses
  epididymitis with early formation of, 234*f*, 234–235
  liver
    amebic, Budd–Chiari syndrome secondary to, 86–87, 86*f*–87*f*
    pylephlebitis and, 30–33, 30*f*–33*f*
  mesenteric, perforated appendicitis with, 176*f*, 176–177
  paracolonic, acute diverticulitis with, 182*f*, 182–183
  pericholecystic, acute cholecystitis with, 110*f*, 110–111
  right renal, diagnosed with power Doppler, 132*f*, 132–133, 134*f*, 134–135
  testicular, partially treated, 242*f*, 242–243
Acquired immunodeficiency syndrome. *See* AIDS
Adenocarcinoma
  bile duct, with carcinomatosis, 106*f*, 106–107
  mucinous cystadenocarcinoma, of pancreas, 116*f*, 116–117
Adenoma
  liver cell, with acute hemorrhage, 20–21, 20*f*–21*f*
  parathyroid, 254*f*, 254–255
  villous, of cecum, presenting as right lower-quadrant pain, 186*f*, 186–187
AIDS-related lymphoma, of liver, 82*f*, 82–83
  flow display with higher frequency, 3, 4*f*
Alcohol ablation, superficial hepatocellular carcinoma treated with, 56–57, 56*f*
Aliasing
  color Doppler, 4, 6*f*
  for differentiation of arteries *vs* veins, 13, 16*f*
  mild, 13, 15*f*
  power Doppler, 8

severe, 13, 15*f*
  simulating flow reversal, 13, 16*f*
Amebic liver abscess, Budd–Chiari syndrome secondary to, 86–87, 86*f*–87*f*
Aneurysms
  mycotic
    of abdominal aorta, 292*f*, 292–293
    of right hepatic artery, secondary to endocarditis, 22–23, 22*f*–23*f*
  portal vein, 50*f*, 50–51
    intrahepatic, cavernous transformation of portal vein with, 90–91, 90*f*–91*f*
    secondary to hepatic vein to portal vein fistula, 38–41, 38*f*–41*f*
  pseudoaneurysms
    femoral artery, color Doppler-directed occlusion of, 284*f*, 284–285
    mycotic, of abdominal aorta, 292*f*, 292–293
    renal artery, bilateral, from unknown angiodysplasia, 130*f*, 130–131
    splenic artery, 272*f*, 272–273
Angiodysplasia, unknown, bilateral renal artery aneurysms from, 130*f*, 130–131
Angle dependency, 263
Aortitis, Takayasu's, involving carotid artery, 290–291, 290*f*–291*f*
Appendicitis
  gangrenous
    with adherent omentum, 188*f*, 188–189
    with marked hyperemia, 174*f*, 174–175
  perforated, with mesenteric abscess and phlegmon, 176*f*, 176–177
  pylephlebitis from, 88*f*, 88–89
Arterial embolization, to splenic artery, with global splenic infarction and pancreatic pseudocyst, 276*f*, 276–277
Arterialization, 283
Arteriovenous fistulas
  common femoral artery to common femoral vein, after cardiac catheterization, 270*f*, 270–271
  of lower pole of kidney, 156*f*, 156–157
  post-renal-biopsy, 154*f*, 154–155
  tissue hum with, 13–16, 17*f*